RICHARD SIMMONS' BETTER BODY BOOK

RICHARD SIMMONS' BETTER BODY BOOK

WARNER BOOKS

A Warner Communications Company

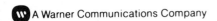 A Warner Communications Company

Printed in the United States of America
First printing: November 1983
10 9 8 7 6 5 4 3 2 1

Library of Congress Cataloging in Publication Data

Simmons, Richard.
   Richard Simmons' better body book

   Includes index.
    1. Reducing exercises.   2. Reducing diets—Recipes.
I. Title.   II. Title: Better body book.
RA781.6.S55   1983   613.7   83-42690
ISBN 0-446-51263-X

Book design by H. Roberts Design

Illustrations copyright © 1983 by Howard Roberts: pages 5, 25, 38, 48, 49, 73, 74, 85, 86, 115, 116, 144, 157, 181, 207, and 218.

There are over two hundred twenty million people in the United States, about seventy million of whom exercise regularly. This book is dedicated to the one hundred fifty million people who aren't exercising, in the hopes that all of them—young, mature, retired, and handicapped—will start taking care of that special gift God has given them—their bodies.

Contents

Acknowledgments

Long before you get your body together
you've got to get your head together,
and that takes friends,
good friends,
who love and understand you.
I got 'em and I thank God for them.
                Thank you
Fred Selleck, Nansey Neiman, Suzy Kalter,
Peggy Ganz, Bill Robbins, Gene Light, Nancy Simmons,
and
Twyla Danielle
for teaching me so very much.

Warning!!!

Please do not leave this book on your coffee table to collect dust. It doesn't like coffee OR dust. And don't just put this book on a shelf with a bunch of other books. It doesn't know how to read.

This *Better Body Book* belongs with your body so it can make your body better. (Now, repeat this sentence five times in a row. See, you're already getting the hang of exercise!)

Basics

My First Time

For most of you this will not be the first exercise book you've ever bought, or received as a gift. (Don't you love it when someone else gives you a book on weight control? I mean, really!)

Personally I could make a down payment on a small foreign car for what I've spent on exercise books. (You too, huh?)

Do you remember the very first exercise book you ever purchased? Now, c'mon, search back through that memory bank of yours. Yep, I thought so. Well, my first was called *Coach Halperin's You Won't Ever Kick Sand in My Face Exercise Manual* by none other than the famous Coach Nathan Halperin. That book was not to be believed—all those guys with crew cuts doing all those stretches right there on the beach. No one in that book even slightly resembled Howdy Doody or Buckwheat. (Or me, either.) It was hard to relate to at first, but that didn't stop me. I began to read the manual, and I am talking about serious reading here. When you take a book into the bathroom with you, it's serious reading.

One day my parents (you remember Len

and Shirl) found the book on my desk, and my mother shouted to my brother, Lenny, "Oh, Lenny dear, you left your exercise book right here on Milton's desk. Better come get it, or he'll give it away."

I ask you, whatever happened to support from the family? Doesn't everyone know that inside every overweight person there's a crew cut just waiting to get out?

Coach Halperin's little manual led to every exercise book I could get my meager biceps on. I hit the libraries, bookstores, and garage sales with dedication and determination. Garage sales were the best. Such bargains I got! I once bought this fabulous book called *Know Your Thighs* (doesn't that title say it all?) by a former Playboy bunny.

Lenny found the book hidden behind the *National Geographic*s and showed it to Dad at the dinner table. Dad punished me by removing the minirefrigerator from my bedroom. Pretty low, huh?

But I didn't quit, not me.

Next came *Uncle Sam Wants Your Body*, a group of boot camp routines compiled by—who else?—the Army, Navy, and Marines in their first joint venture since D day. This book was filled with sweat and—you guessed it—more crew cuts.

I kept looking for some easy way, some shortcut to all the physical activity that looked so boring. I finally found it. When my mother would go into the kitchen to cook one of her simple seven-course meals, I would sneak into Mom and Dad's room and hunt around for Mom's copy of *Modern Screen*. Heaven, it was heaven. All these movie stars would go on for pages, talking about how they kept in shape. And then, in the back, there were all these booklets you could send away for that promised **Overnight Flat Stomach** and **Fantastic Arms in Ten Days.** Naturally I sent away for all these. I would do a few of the exercises—you know, a leg lift here, a leg lift there—and then I'd give up, because, well, don't you ever hear this little voice that tells you to quit?

For years I was a searcher. I'd buy anything that gave me the slightest bit of hope. Then one day I realized you could be a looker or a doer. The very word *exercise* got to be a turnoff. When I starved for two and a half months, I refused to exercise at all. (Except for a little walking. I mean, when you starve, who has the energy to do anything but use the remote control button for the television?) I've got to be honest with you. My body looked better heavy than it did after losing all that weight without exercising. I looked like a chocolate malted-milk ball after someone sucked the insides out of it.

I was a shrunken version of my former self. Where there had been fat, I was left with droopy skin and stretch marks. That's when I remembered some of those exercise books from my youth and the magic words about toning. Having a thin body isn't of much value, physically or socially, if it isn't toned and tight. I know that when you imagine yourself thin, you also imagine yourself shapely and gorgeous. There's only one way to accomplish that goal: exercise. I think that most people lose some weight, take a look at how awful they look, get discouraged, and go off their food plans. Then they gain back all the weight they have lost and feel depressed.

It's easy to give up, I know that. It's easy to throw a book like this across the room. (That's a good exercise for the upper arm. Now, repeat twenty times, each side.) It's easy to give in to excuses and that little voice inside you that says it's hopeless.

However, the best things in life aren't easy. It's hard to get down on your mat each day; it's hard to do those push-ups and those sit-ups. But, honest to God, you can do it. I did it. I know you can.

This book is a virtual encyclopedia of the body. If you pay attention and learn what's in this book and then apply it to that body of yours, you will have a better body. If you add to that a sensible food plan, you will lose weight and have a slimmer, firmer body at the same time. I don't care how many times you've tried before—I know you can do it this time. Read this book, use that head of yours, and work on that body every day, and your life, as well as your body, will change.

When you finish this book, you will have one of the biggest choices of your life to make. You can choose to be one of the one hundred fifty million people who don't exercise, one of those millions of people who keep buying and selling their diet and exercise books at garage sales. OR you can be a winner. You can use this book as your lifetime guide. Everything you need to have a better body is right here in your hands. The choice is yours.

I'm rooting for you.

A Short History of Exercise

In the beginning there was Adam and Eve. At first they were doing great, because they worked real hard each day and ate plenty of natural foods and hardly ever had a Coke, so their teeth were pretty good and their bodies were firm. They never really had to worry much about exercise, because their life-style was pretty rigorous and staying alive was exercise enough. Then came the fateful day when Eve decided to make Waldorf salad, and the rest is history. They were banished from the Garden of Eden, without so much as a car or a guidebook, and had to go jogging around the world in search of paradise lost. I don't need to tell you that this was how jogging was invented.

While several sports evolved during the biblical ages (Noah taught long-distance swimming to everyone he couldn't take on the Ark; Daniel was a champion body builder and a wrestler long before he happened about the lion's den, etc.), the Greeks really made exercise what it is today. The first Olympics was held in 776 B.C. (this is for real, I am not making this up, guys), which was, in case you don't have your Week At A Glance handy, one hell of a long time ago. The Olympics happens to be, in fact, one of the few enterprises begun by man to last such a long time. (Even Christmas looks like a newcomer compared to the Olympics.)

Winning the Olympics (which was held every four years, even then) was such a big deal that kings competed with commoners to bring home the gold—the greatest honor any Greek could win—and those who took home an olive branch (this was after olives but before gold medals) became national heroes. Musicians sang their praises, magazines tattled their secrets, and sculptors carved their strength and beauty into marble. Since this was also before air pollution, the marble lasted throughout the centuries and passed on to mankind the model body form. Thereafter men and women throughout the ages tried to attain the same form as those long-dead heroes.

It was Marco Polo who brought the sport of polo to Europe and eventually to Ralph Lauren. You see, Marco happened to note that Kublai Khan's soldiers spent off-hours (when not plundering and looting) on horseback with golf clubs with which they knocked back and forth to each other the severed heads of former enemies. While Marco had to do some modifying of the sport to make it acceptable in European circles, he did come around to the notion of using a ball as a replacement for the head, and thus the game bearing his name became the sport of kings and is still played today wherever people are rich.

Henry VIII knew well the connection between exercise and weight control. When a bad leg forced him to quit his aerobic dance class, he began to overeat and grew to obesity (that's polite for fat). Exercise for royalty didn't become popularized until the reign of Louis XIV. The women in the court took to exercising as a solution to the biggest fashion problem of the day. Until then genteel ladies were to exercise only their tongues in gossip, their fingers in needlework, or their palms in card games. But when hairstyles became so cumbersome that entire shipyards were constructed in curled and teased tendrils, a woman had to have a strong set of neck and shoulder muscles to be able to hold her head up high. So it came to pass that the most fashionable women did exercises in their boudoirs until noon and then continued with isometrics once their hairdressers arrived at one. This is also how waists were kept to the prescribed sixteen inches and chests were able to match the fashionable flatness of the era. A few Louises later Marie Antoinette was far too busy worrying about her waistline ("let them eat cake," she said, since she was on a strict food plan) to do shoulder rounds, which might have helped save her from a pain in the neck.

It was the real people, not the kings, who came up with most of the other sports: Robin Hood and his merry band of men invented archery; Christopher Columbus, on his first trip to the Caribbean, discovered the islands of Cuba and Aruba and took up Arubacizing; Tom Sawyer invented fencing on a summer day; and Paul Revere made horse racing a respectable sport. Even mobsters have played their part in the history of exercise. Al Capone invented racquetball!

And you thought Jack LaLanne invented the whole thing.

The Three Stooges Meet the Invisible Man

Quick, name a body type.
Fat.
Thin.
Obese.
Wrong.

You may have had a body all your life, but I don't think you know too much of this scientific stuff. (I know, it used to put me to sleep, too.)

Despite the fact that God created all men (and women) equal, there seems to be a big difference in exactly how some peoples' bodies work. Some people retain water and gain weight that is mostly fluid. Some people can put on weight, to the tune of five pounds or so, at one meal. There are people who can't gain weight no matter how hard they try, and they even have trouble putting on muscle. But just you remember—a thin body doesn't mean a good body. You can be sleek and still be totally out of shape.

You have a natural body type (usually inherited, so you can put the blame on Mame) that will influence the direction you take in reshaping your body. You are either an ectomorph, a mesomorph, or an endomorph.

Endomorphs

I'll start with them, because I think that by birth I am an endomorph. Endomorphs are a little bit shorter and a little bit rounder, naturally, than everyone else. I'm not rounder now, because—just as I've said you can—I've redesigned my body. But I was born short and fat, my brother, Lenny, leans toward the short and plump, and so does my mother. (My Dad was skinny. Endomorphs gain fat more easily than other people and may actually be weak despite their bulky size. It's especially hard for an endomorph to shape up and stay in shape, so he needs to know that he's fighting a body type and must be determined to win. In endomorphs the fat cells gang together in bands or ribbons that thread themselves around specific parts of the body to make staying in shape especially hard—but not impossible! It's real easy for the endomorph to quit while on a food and exercise program and say, "I was meant to be fat." That's just an excuse. Many superb athletes are endomorphs, and if I can end up looking like a pixie, so can anyone else.

Mesomorphs

Robert Redford is probably a mesomorph, and Arnold Schwarzenegger and Superman and even Tarzan. Mesomorphs are naturally strong, agile, well built, and gorgeous. Their biggest problem is that if they don't work out regularly, they can gain a little paunch, get hippy (they are the ones who believe the most in spot reducing), or have plain old weak bodies, because they haven't kept themselves in prime condition. I have the

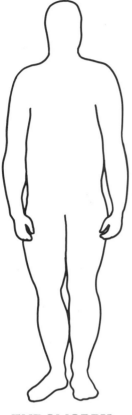

ENDOMORPH

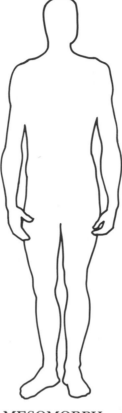

MESOMORPH

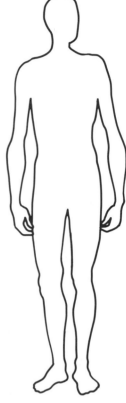

ECTOMORPH

least sympathy for mesomorphs, because their bodies were created as perfectly as a piece of fine machinery, and they have only themselves to blame if they get winded climbing stairs, can't jog around the block, or look like the Thanksgiving turkey incarnate by Super Bowl time. To not keep a body like this in shape is a sin. (And I went to Catholic school, so I know a lot about sin!)

Ectomorphs

These guys are the worst. Naturally tall and thin, the ectomorph actually has trouble putting on fat. But don't hate them, because most ectomorphs think that because they are thin, they don't need to exercise. As a result they are weak, have poor heart power, and may be low on endurance. Ectomorphs are the type that often look weak and fragile and may be ready to faint after half an exercise

class. Talk about your ninety-pound weakling! They have backaches during pregnancy because they're so out of shape, and they couldn't begin to make it halfway up Mount Everest, even with a whole team of Sherpas to shove them.

Knowing your own body type will help you to reshape your figure because you will be able to set your mental gauge according to how difficult the task will be.

- Endomorphs will be challenged—but don't give up!
- Ectomorphs will have a hard time (we'll try to be sympathetic).
- Mesomorphs will have the best results.

To help you get the hang of figuring out a body type, try this little quiz. All you have to do is fill in the type of body you think these famous people have (or had). The answers are on page 6, so no cheating.

1. Cheryl Tiegs _____
2. Raquel Welch _____
3. Sophia Loren _____
4. Dustin Hoffman _____
5. Kareem Abdul-Jabbar _____
   (Everyone's entitled to a few real easy ones, don'tcha think?)
6. Elizabeth Taylor _____
7. Susan Anton _____
8. Mahalia Jackson _____
9. Ronald Reagan _____
10. Shelley Winters _____
11. Davy Crockett (or Fess Parker, whichever you think of first) _____
12. Abraham Lincoln _____
13. Diana Ross _____
14. Juanita Wasserman _____
    (Okay, this is a tricky one.)
15. Princess Diana _____
    (Another difficult one, so I'll give you a clue: She's not an ectomorph.)

Answers

1. Cheryl Tiegs is an ectomorph.
2. Raquel Welch is a mesomorph.
3. Sophia Loren is an endomorph.
4. Dustin Hoffman is an endomorph.
5. Kareem Abdul-Jabbar is an ectomorph.
6. Elizabeth Taylor is an endomorph.
7. Susan Anton is an ectomorph.
8. Mahalia Jackson is an endomorph.
9. Ronald Reagan is a mesomorph.
10. Shelley Winters is an endomorph.
11. Davy Crockett was a mesomorph.
12. Abraham Lincoln was an ectomorph.
13. Diana Ross is a mesomorph.
14. Juanita Wasserman is an endomorph.
15. Princess Diana is a tall mesomorph.

The Truth About Exercise

There are two things about exercise that I think everyone should know before starting an exercise program. Most people will string you along and give you a big list of reasons why you should exercise (you know that list: You won't have a heart attack, you'll fit into a bikini, you'll live longer, you'll have more energy) without telling you any of the nitty-gritty—less-than-life-and-death things that really do count.

So here it is, folks, the honest to goodness list of things you can count on.

Number One: You'll Be Sore

The first time I went to exercise class the paramedics had to come and take me home.

Oh, I kept up with the class all right, and I had a great time getting involved and being enthusiastic. No one could say I didn't keep up with the Joneses' leg lifts. But by the end of the hour I could hardly even pant. I needed a team of firemen, two dalmatians, and the paramedics just to get me into bed. My legs were wobbling, my hands looked like they had played "Heart and Soul" on the piano for twenty hours straight, and I had one of those Walkman headaches. (I play mine on nine, how about you?) I didn't go back to class for a week and when I did, I was sore all over again.

I stopped going to class for six months. I remembered the soreness, and it was a great excuse for staying away. I could blame it on the teacher (she was too hard), the wood floors (they were too hard)—even on the bossa nova. Finally I went back. I held back and was determined to stretch out my muscles slowly and to build up strength. I walked out of class on my own two feet and felt quite proud. I went to work that day and the next with a smug feeling of accomplishment. On the second day after the class I felt intense throbbing in every muscle in my body. I did not have a charley horse in my leg—I had a charley horse in every available space in my body. I was one big stable. And I used that as an excuse not to go to class for several more months.

If your body is out of shape, if you haven't been in a regular exercise program in the last year, if you have trouble walking up a flight of stairs without huffing and puffing (unless you are wearing an oxygen mask—and that's cheating), you are going to be sore when you start to exercise. So remember:

• Start out carefully and build up gradually. If you feel sore enough to feel the pull but not too sore to get around without a wheelchair, you are the right amount of sore.
• Do not try to keep up with a class that is in better shape than you are, especially if you are overweight.
• Push your body to do a little more each day. Don't do a lot and then fall backward. Stopping and starting on programs causes soreness.
• If an exercise hurts while you are doing it (as opposed to right after or later), stop immediately.
• If something hurts, after class take time to ask the instructor if you are doing the exercise correctly. A boo-boo may harm your body.
• If you do too much and become sore despite my warnings and your best intentions, do not take to bed and quit the world. Warm showers or baths, whirlpool treatments, or hot tub soaks may help you feel better. Continue minimal stretching exercises unless you have specific pain. DON'T DO ANYTHING THAT HURTS, but do maintain movement when possible. Massage may help, or maybe ice.

Because you are sore, you will want to use it as an excuse:

• "I can't go back to class today, I'll die."
• "If I exercise while I am sore, I'll make things worse."
• "I've tried exercising, but my body rejects it; when my body talks, I have to listen."

Try listening to me instead. Being sore tells you how much your body needs exercise. Soreness means the exercise is working. You aren't a Barbie or a Ken doll. If you stretch your arm a bit, it won't fall off. Learn how much your body can handle each day.

Number Two: You'll Think of Excuses

I don't know why it is, but more people turn into babies when it comes time to exercise. I've just never seen anything like it. The craziest excuses come out of people's mouths; the lamest reasons not to go to class cross people's brains.

It takes about a year of steady exercise for your body to be hooked on it. Once you've gotten past the first six months, it's easier for you and you look forward to the exercise and miss it if something gets in the way. But until that time, until you go over the hump, you will baby yourself and come up with the most amazing excuses for not exercising.

• "My nails are wet."
• "I've got my period."
• "It's raining outside."
• "It would be dangerous in my delicate condition."
• "I need my sleep more than I need to exercise." (This one works a lot of the time.)
• "There's no place to go near my house." (I don't know why they don't have aerobics classes in McDonald's, they have them just about everyplace else.)
• "I don't have time."

The I-don't-have-time bunch are always my favorite, because every Sunday night you find them glued in front of their television sets, watching Morley Safer and *60 Minutes*. They've got time for a show, but they don't have sixty minutes for their own bodies! I mean, you have time for the things that are important, and if you have such low self-esteem that your body isn't important to you, that's your problem.

I too used to fluctuate in my dedication to my exercise routine. I'd go to class real steady for a while, then skip a day. The day turned into a week, then a month. Pretty soon it was months before I'd done anything, and I had to deal with guilt galore before I got to class again. (Usually one look at my body in a full-length mirror did the trick.)

Once I was out to dinner, and I bumped into my aerobics teacher, who asked me why I hadn't been in class lately.

"My parents are in town," I told her, "and I've been sick . . . real sick. . . . In fact, this is my first night out of bed in a month . . . that's why my parents had to come into town . . . in case I died. . . . I pulled something, you know, but I'll be back in class tomorrow. I promise."

She interrupted me as I was swearing I would appear.

"Listen, you want a healthy-looking body, right? Well, it's not easy. If it was easy, don't you think every person out there would have a great-looking body? You just think about that."

So I pass her words of wisdom on to you.

I still get sore.

I still think of a stray excuse I haven't used before.

But in the end I go to class and I work out in my home gym, because I know the bottom line. My bottom line. There are no good excuses. I still get sore. I am sore because I push my body a little further every day. And I guess I'm proud to be sore.

The Better Body Quiz

Since you don't seem to know very much about your body, before you start shaking it out and giving yourself a hernia, let's see exactly what you know and don't know and where you should begin your pursuit of the new you. It doesn't do you much good to jump in and exercise if you're going to fall out the next day due to sore, tired muscles or torn, broken ligaments. (Okay, you can't really break a ligament.) Take this quiz and find out if you should be a beginner, an intermediate, or an advanced exerciser. Then if you have special circumstances, like pregnancy or a lot of extra pounds, see pages 267 and 253.

Answer honestly. The fate of your figure is in your hands.

1. **The last time I seriously exercised was:**
   a. yesterday.
   b. within the last year.
   c. Who can remember that far back?

2. **The shape my body is in right now is:**
   a. admirable.
   b. a bit heavier than I would like; I must take off five to ten pounds.
   c. embarrassing.

3. **If I was to bend over right now I could:**
   a. touch my toes.
   b. touch somewhere between my toes and my knees.
   c. see the dust on the floor.

4. **The amount of weight I need to lose is:**
   a. less than five pounds.
   b. between five and fifteen pounds.
   c. over fifteen pounds.

5. My idea of warming up is:
   a. stretching and breathing to get my muscles ready for action.
   b. putting on a sweater.
   c. turning the thermostat up to 75 degrees.

6. My diaphragm is important for:
   a. breathing.
   b. burping.
   c. birth control.

7. Besides my exercise program, I am also involved in sports:
   a. at least twice a week, maybe more.
   b. most weekends.
   c. I like to watch.

8. My life-style is:
   a. active.
   b. sedentary—I don't get as much exercise as I would like.
   c. inactive—La Blob—I do not exercise.

9. Laps are:
   a. the number of times I swim across the pool.
   b. the people who live in Lapland.
   c. nice for sitting on.

10. Lisa Lyons is:
   a. the world's leading female body builder.
   b. the actress who played Lolita.
   c. a girl in Mrs. Clines's nursery school class.

11. When I walk up a flight of stairs or two:
   a. I feel no pain or distraction.
   b. I feel somewhat winded and sorry I didn't take the elevator.
   c. I feel like fainting; I am huffing and puffing and have pains in my chest.

12. The size of the clothes I wear is:
   a. the same as it was since high school or college.
   b. the same size, more or less.
   c. no one else's business.

13. A good exercise program should include:
   a. three different types of exercise: for flexibility, the heart, and the muscles.
   b. great music.
   c. a lot of cute guys.

14. After exercise I feel:
   a. a real high.
   b. great. Why don't I do this more often?
   c. closer to death.

15. My body:
   a. is only as good as I keep it.
   b. needs a little work.
   c. is a disaster area.

To Score:

Give yourself one point for every C answer, three points for every B answer, and five points for every A answer. The lower your score, the worse shape you are in!

If Your Score Is 15–35

Pitiful. The only thing I can congratulate you on is the courage to tell the truth. You haven't exercised in years, you aren't even familiar with the latest exercise terms, and you have been neglecting, I said neglecting, your body. You are a BEGINNER, no question about it. And if you are fifty pounds or more overweight, you belong in an OVER-WEIGHTER class (see page 253).

If Your Score Is 36–59

Well, that's not too bad. You are at least in the aware category and know what you should and shouldn't be doing. You're probably just lacking a little bit in motivation. Just how long have you needed to take off five to ten pounds, huh? If you've exercised in the last year, but not in the last couple of months, spend three or four weeks with the BEGINNER program and then proceed to INTERMEDIATE. If you do exercise more than four hours a week, give BEGINNER a week, then proceed to INTERMEDIATE.

If Your Score Is Over 60

Congratulations, you are in tune with your body and your self. If you want a job on my show, give me a call. Proceed to INTERMEDIATE.

One Day at a Time

No, this isn't a review of your favorite television show. It's a reminder. Before you begin to work on having a better body, give yourself a break. Don't make outrageous demands on yourself. Don't set goals for weight loss, size of clothing, figure measurements, or anything else. Take it one day at a time.

If you have the wrong expectations, you will disappoint yourself. You'll get frustrated and you'll quit. And you won't have a better body—inside or outside.

It takes about a year to really get in shape. It takes a lifetime to stay in shape. Do a little a day, every day. Begin slowly. Almost everyone should start with the BEGINNER program. Your goal is to do only a little bit more each day. It's a personal goal and it's for you alone. You won't get results if you don't stick to this plan. Once you see some results, you'll be motivated to go for more. So don't blow it by being a pig. Slow and steady wins the race.

This is the only exercise book that offers several programs so you can tailor them to your needs. Don't be embarrassed to start out as a beginner. Be proud that each day you do a little more. Be proud that eventually you will be ready to move into INTERMEDIATE. This book is as hard or as easy as your body needs. Once you've lost weight and gotten your figure where you want it to be, you'll maintain your new great shape with the ADVANCED program. But get there slowly and enjoy your progress. Every day you will be a better you.

Before You Begin

Have you ever noticed that every diet or food book and every exercise book you buy (and I know you've bought plenty of them, just like I have) has a sentence in it someplace—be it in little print or big block letters—that tells you not to exercise until you have had a medical checkup?

Why, you ask yourself, do you have to get a physical? Why pee in a bottle, run on a treadmill, get electrodes stuck to you, take this test and that test, and spend maybe two hundred dollars?

I'll tell you why.

So you don't die. We've all heard stories about youngish men who drop dead on the tennis court, or people who are doing their best to stay healthy and meet up all too suddenly with the Angel of Death, who doesn't even wear good jogging shoes. Let's face it—it's extremely frightening.

A medical checkup with a test or two may cost a hundred dollars, but it beats falling over on the curbside because you thought jogging in a marathon was something you really could do.

Safe is always better than sorry.

So don't get frightened and don't get scared—be sensible.

Don't say "Yeah, yeah, I ought to do that." Pick up your phone, make an appointment for the physical, and do it—spend the money. You've spent more than that on diet and fitness books over the last decade, haven't you?

Do this right. Don't be sorry. End of story.

If It Were Easy, Everyone Would Have a Great Body

1

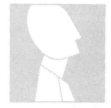

Face and Neck

Let's Face It

The face is one of the trickiest parts of your body. It can do many things and make many expressions. I personally have been practicing expression making since I was three years old and have found a variety of uses for my nose, lips, mouth, teeth, tongue, and eyes in trying to scare the living daylights out of my brother, Lenny.

Now I practice my same rubber face techniques so I don't scare myself when I look in the mirror. Exercising the face muscles will not make them wrinkle more, it will keep the muscles under your skin tight and help prevent the face lift you hope you won't need. If you do some face-saving exercises every day, you can retard the aging process. You can't restore missing tone, but you can prevent sagging before it starts.

Fight Aging with Exercise

There's no question about it. Exercising will help you fight the aging process. I've seen thirty-year-olds with the bodies of seventy-five-year-olds. I've seen sixty-year-olds who can pass for forty, easily. You are only as old as you let your body be. True, there are many body changes that bring on some of the symptoms of old age, but medical science is working on these.

If you eat wisely, maintain an even weight for most of your life, avoid smoking, drinking, and drug abuse, AND exercise regularly, you will live a lot longer and a lot better. I mean, what's the use of living extra years if they aren't going to be active, good years? If you take care of yourself NOW and EXER-

CISE, I promise you, they will be good years.

One of the areas where you will see the reward of daily exercise is in your face and neck. Eating three meals a day is not my idea of giving your face muscles a workout—no matter how much you are chewing. The face may be expressive, but you have to take the time to do a series of exercises to use the muscles that make up your face if you want to keep them from sagging over the years. Why worry about the expense of a face lift when you can prevent yourself from needing one! You've heard of preventive medicine? Well, here's a real way to look younger, look better, and prevent the need for plastic surgery.

F1 *Richard's Vowels*

Position: standing in front of a mirror so you can see your muscles working.

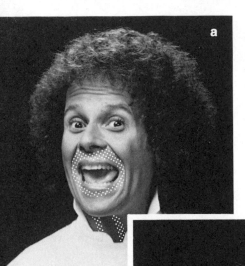

1. **Pronounce each of the vowels (AEIOU) slowly while exaggerating them.**

2. **Open your mouth wide and really move those muscles.**

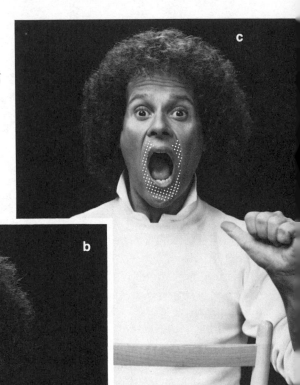

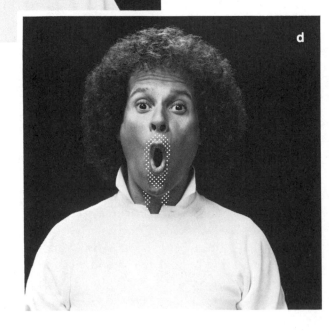

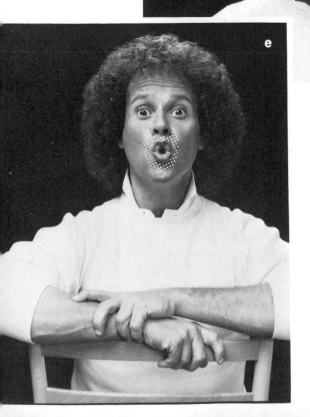

F2 Side Wipes

Position: *in front of a mirror.*

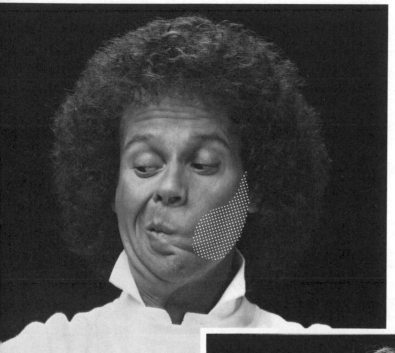

1. Contort your face in a pout first to the right, then to the left.

2. It's not unusual for one side to be easier than the other.

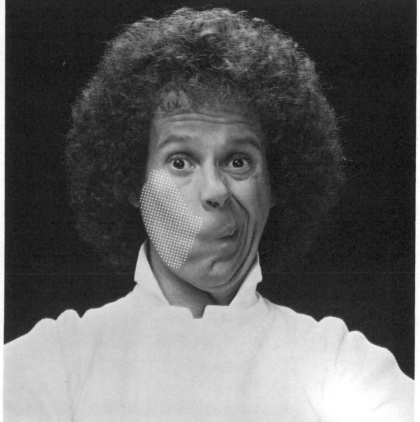

F3 Chews

Position: in front of a mirror.

1. **Neck up, smile a big Miss America smile.**

2. **Chew the air without grinding your teeth.**

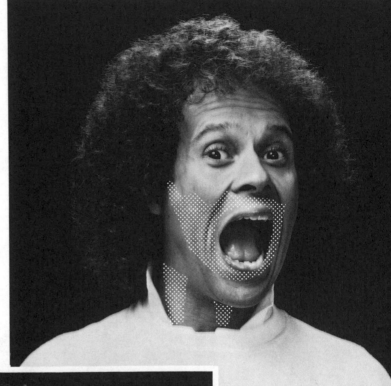

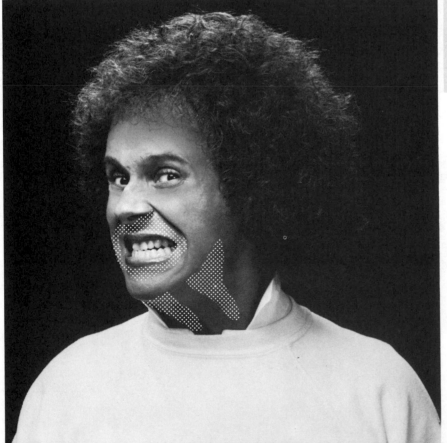

F4 *Pout and Drops*

Position: *in front of a mirror.*

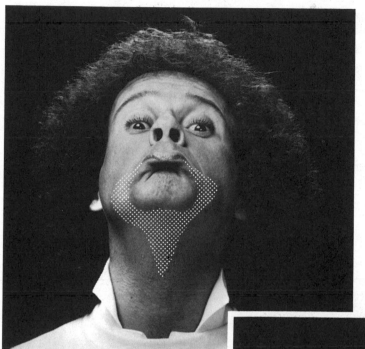

1. Put your head back, keeping your shoulders down.

2. Form a pout, then drop it.

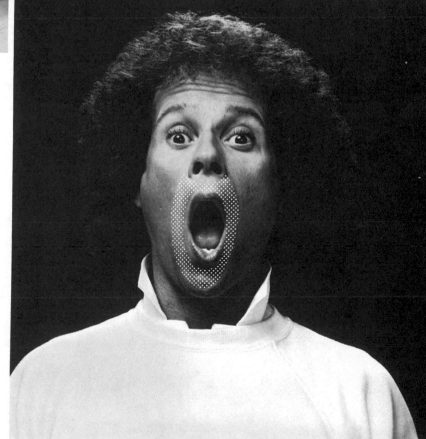

F5 *Tongue Extensions*

Position: *in front of a mirror.*

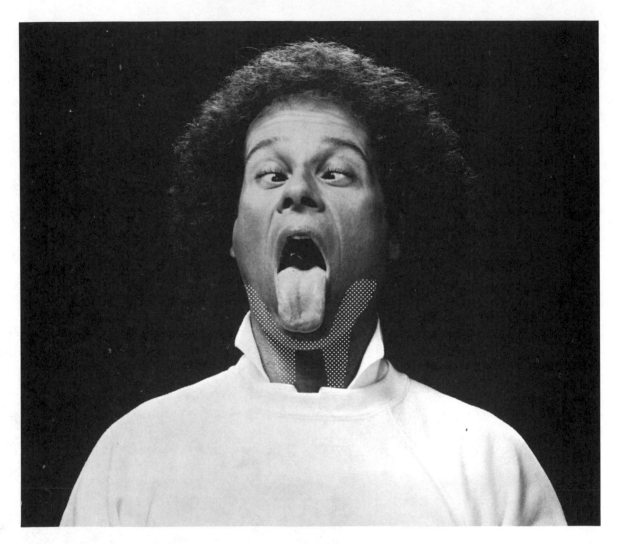

1. Stick your tongue out as far as you can, with a downward thrust to your chin.

2. If you can touch your chest with your tongue, you've done too many.

F6 Kissy Kissys

Position: in front of a mirror.

1. **Pucker up.**

2. **Release, repeat, etc.**

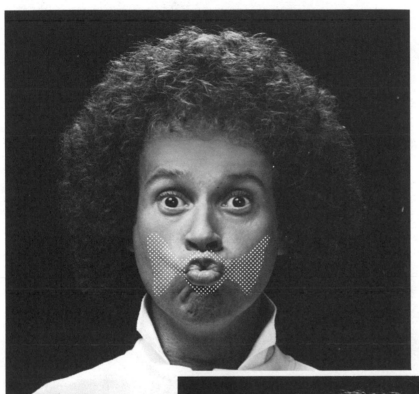

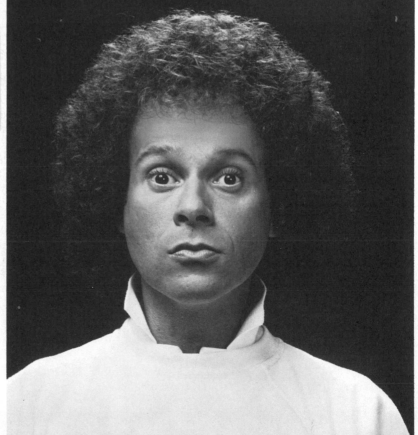

F7 Frown Ups

Position: in front of a mirror.

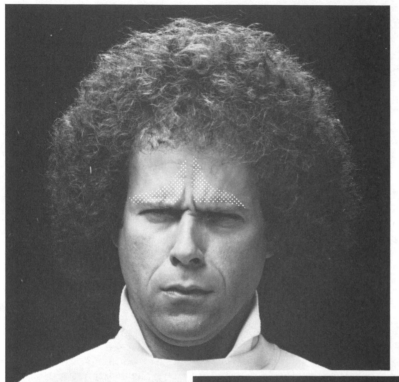

1. Crinkle your face into a frown.

2. Open your eyes in amazement.

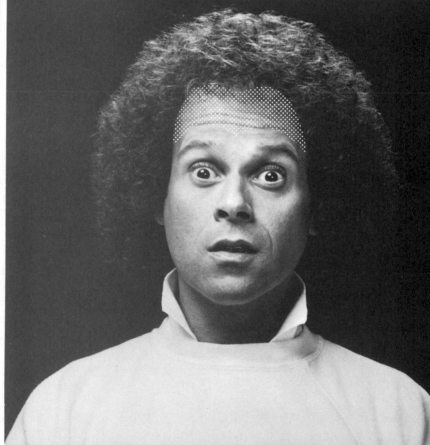

F8 Blinks

Position: in front of a mirror.

1. **Exaggerate blinking, with your eyes crunched tight.**

2. **Open eyes wide, looking up.**

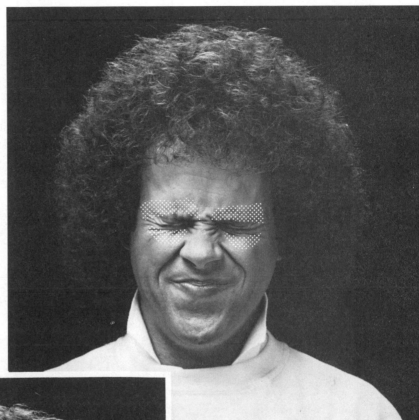

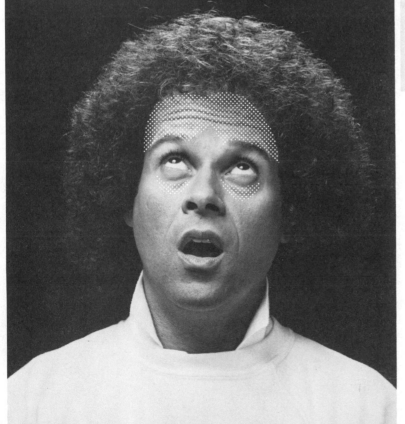

F9 Side Winks

Position: in front of a mirror.

1. Frown and then wink on right side.

2. Frown again and wink on left side.

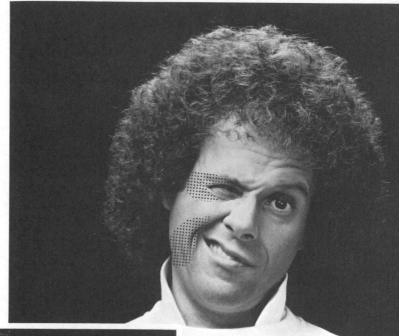

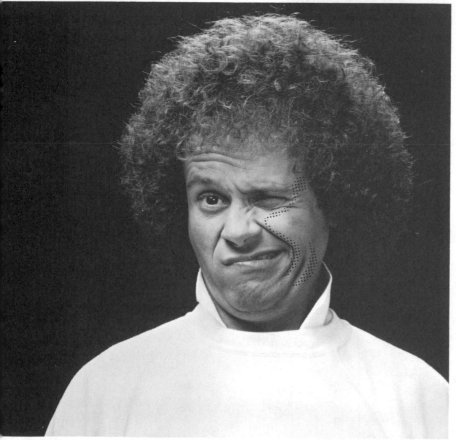

The Neck

The skull (that's medicalese for head bone) rests on top of seven little bones called the cervical vertebrae. (That won't be on the quiz.) The very first of these vertebrae in your neck is called the atlas. It doesn't shrug, but it is responsible for making your head tip. The other six vertebrae make the neck bend. Both of these are important movements in kissing, thus the term *necking*.

This simple feat of engineering makes your neck one of the most flexible parts of your body. The neck is also one of your body's most vital and vulnerable areas. Even the skin around your neck is more sensitive than most of the other skin that covers your body. The vertebrae that make up your neck are smaller than the ones in your back, and the ligaments that hold them in place are much weaker than the ones in, say, your lower back—which is the key to your neck's flexibility and the reason why it is so fragile.

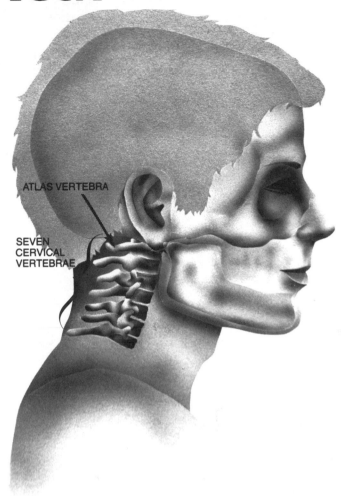

THE NECK

Neck Talk

Because of it's location, the neck is one of the main target areas of stress pain. At the slightest suggestion of tension or fear the delicate muscles in the neck clench up. Once they tighten, you feel it immediately.

You can spot tension in the neck by observing any of these signs in yourself or someone else:

• Turtle Syndrome—or a "bull neck." The neck is pulled in as close to the body as possible. At the same time the shoulders are raised, so that the neck just about disappears.

• Camel Syndrome. The neck is stuck way out in front of the body like a camel trying to win the race to the oasis by a nose. The head is pushed forward, out of alignment with the rest of the body.

• Bullfrog Syndrome. The muscles or veins in the neck stick out or twitch.

• Millstone Syndrome. The teeth are ground, while either awake or asleep, or the jaw is clamped as a nervous habit.

• Pisa Syndrome. The head leans to one side all the time.

If you suffer from any of these problems, relax (I know: easier said than done) and shake it on out. Neck tension and stress will only make the rest of your body uncomfortable, lead to more serious trouble, and cause fatigue and grouchiness. Do a few head rolls and loosen up.

Any of these things can make you tighten up and will cause what is traditionally known as a pain in the neck:

- hunching in front of the TV, over a book, or at a desk
- crummy posture
- the way you drive
- fear
- a draft (That's why Mom told you to button your coat and wear a scarf.)
- flu and colds
- emotions
- arthritis
- looking over the top of your glasses
- sleeping in a crazy position
- disk disease
- headache.

Neck pain may be specific to your neck and may be something that will go away in a matter of hours, or could be related to a problem in your arms, shoulders, back, or chest. If your neck pain travels to another part of your body, get a doctor's opinion. If you suffer from stiff neck, treat it yourself with first rest, then exercise. NEVER exercise a neck that hurts. Maintain a range of motion without pain, but don't push yourself to superhuman tasks. Your neck should move about 90 degrees to each side, 30 degrees backward and forward, and you should be able to touch your chin to your chest without pain.

According to *Shōgun*, from which I learned everything I know about Japanese culture (I love Richard Chamberlain), the Japanese have long considered the back of the neck to be very sexy. It is true that the neck is a sensitive area, because it has so many nerves and an excellent supply of blood, and a light touch at the neck is considered arousing by many. However, the neck is such a vulnerable area that people are often worried about being strangled by a too-tight grasp there. This fear is natural and is difficult to unlearn, thus neck play must be gentle to be effective.

Can you do these things?

If not, why not?

CAN YOU DO THIS?

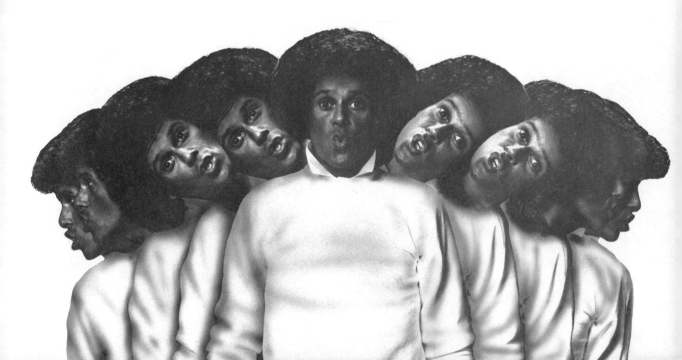

F10 Neck Stretches

Position: standing, shoulders back, neck straight.

1. Using your best military posture, stretch your neck forward, touching your chin *almost* to your chest, then stretch your neck backward (without leaning your body back).

2. Do this exercise slowly, stretching out those stiff muscles. Don't jerk your head back and forth too quickly.

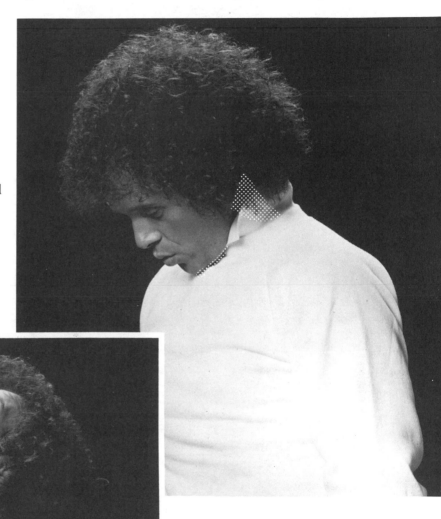

F11 Side to Sides

Position: standing, shoulders back, neck held high.

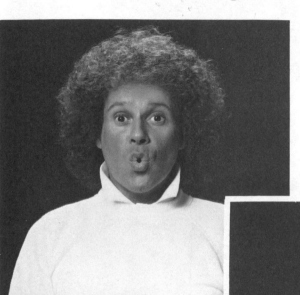

1. Plant your feet slightly apart and stretch your neck first to the left, then to the right.

2. Don't bring your shoulders up to meet your neck when you do this exercise—that's cheating.

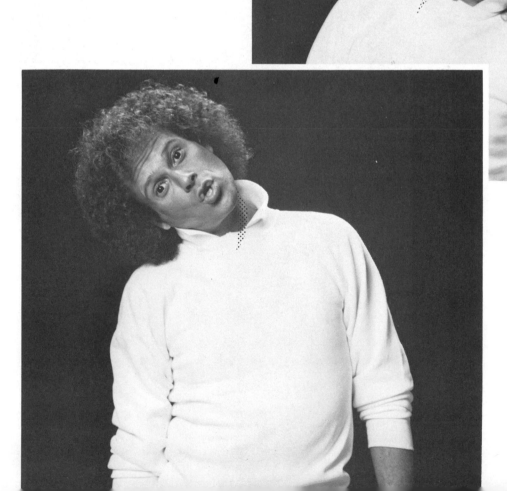

F12 Neck Turns

Position: standing, shoulders back, neck held high.

1. Look straight ahead.

2. Turn head side to side without twisting your shoulders.

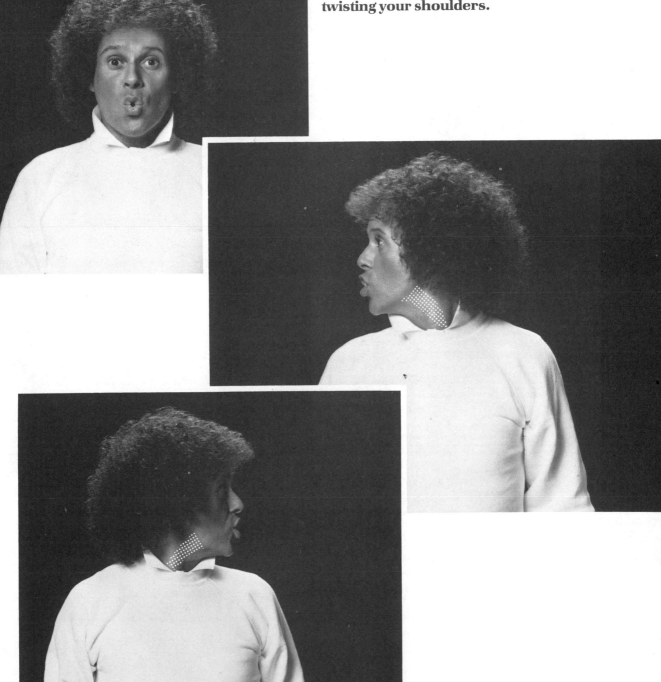

F13 Head Rolls

Position: standing, shoulders relaxed.

1. In a smooth, continuous motion roll your head all the way around toward the right, making a complete circle, then reverse.

2. Your shoulders should be dropped.

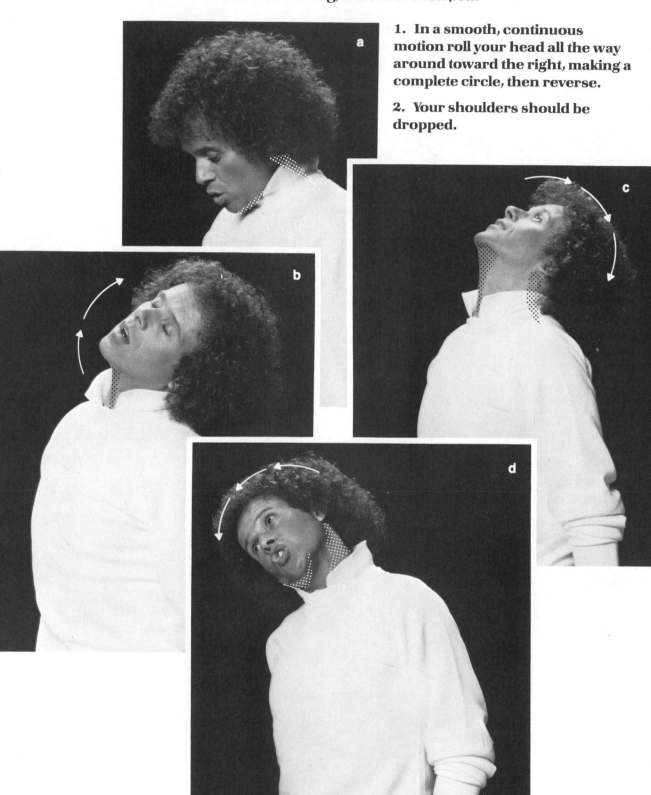

F14 Side Neck Pulls

Position: standing, feet slightly apart.

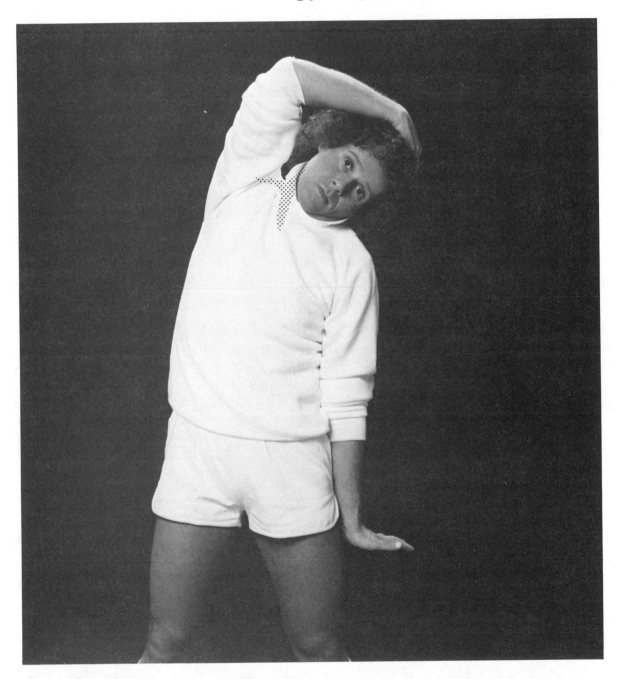

1. **Raise your right arm over your head, bending at the elbow, letting your hand droop over your head to grab your left ear.**

2. **Flex your left hand and push down gently.**

3. **Alternate sides.**

F15 Forward Neck Pulls

Position: standing, feet slightly apart.

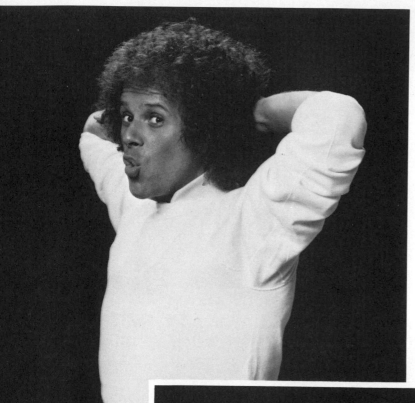

1. Lace fingers behind your head (not your neck). Elbows are pointing out.

2. Gently curl your head down toward your chest. The weight of your arms will pull down on your neck.

3. DO NOT BOUNCE! Just hold that position until you feel relaxed.

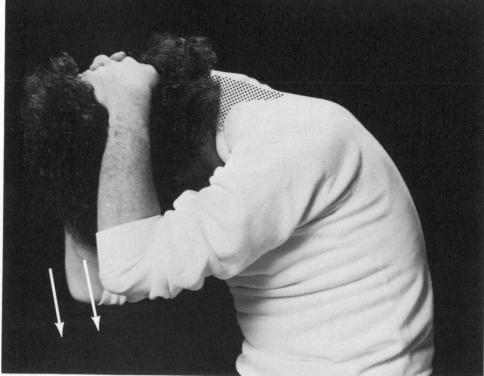

F16 Neck Resistance—Up

Position: standing, feet slightly apart.

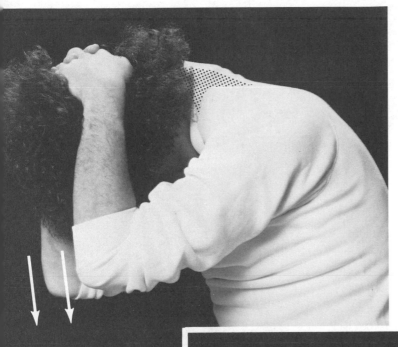

1. Your fingers are clasped behind your head (not your neck). Elbows are pointing straight out.

2. Gently curl your head down toward your chest. The weight of your arms will pull down on your neck.

3. Try to raise your head up as your arms pull down.

4. DO NOT BOUNCE!

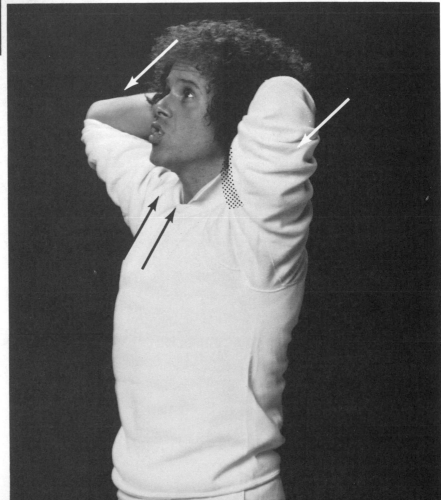

F17 Neck Resistance—Down

Position: standing, feet slightly apart.

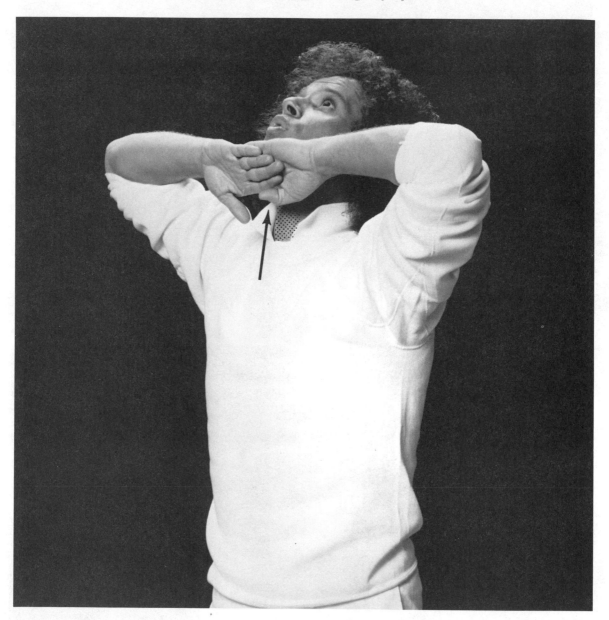

1. This time your hands are clasped under your chin, with your head leaning back.

2. Elbows are at right angles.

3. Your hands try to push your chin up as your chin pushes down. Do not move your jaw.

F18 Side Resistance

Position: standing, feet slightly apart.

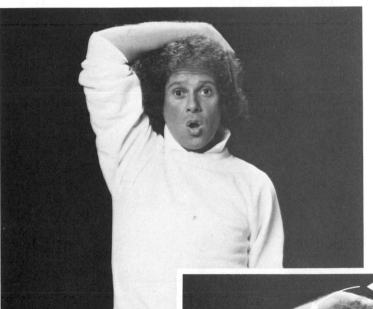

1. Reach your right hand up over your head, elbow bent, and touch your left ear.

2. Flex your left hand and push down.

3. Try to lift your head up as your hand pushes down.

4. Alternate sides.

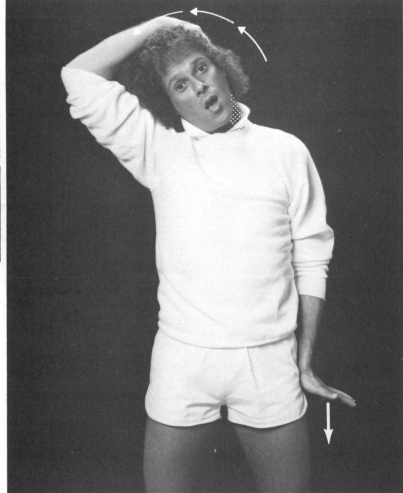

The Quiz

You thought I was kidding when I said there would be a quiz, didn't you? Well, the joke's on you. You have fifteen minutes to bone up. Then let's see just how seriously you're taking this new, improved body business. This is true/false, and no cheating, please.

		T	F
1.	The atlas of your neck was created by Rand McNally.	T	F
2.	Your neck should move 90 degrees to each side.	T	F
3.	The sternomastoid muscle is used in the rotation of the neck.	T	F
4.	Exercise can and will affect how your face ages.	T	F
5.	Bad posture can cause serious neck pain.	T	F
6.	You can get a stiff neck from a cold draft.	T	F
7.	If you have neck pain, exercise immediately.	T	F
8.	Arthritis sufferers often have neck pain.	T	F
9.	Exercise can help ease tension in the neck.	T	F
10.	The neck is one of the body's most vulnerable areas.	T	F

Answers

(I'm not printing them upside down, because I don't want you to strain your neck reading them.)

1. F   2. F   3. T   4. T   5. T   6. T   7. F   8. T   9. T   10. T

2

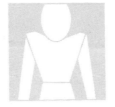

Shoulders

Sister Mary Justine
Explains It All to You

"Why did God create shoulders?" I asked Sister Mary Justine, my fifth grade science teacher. "I thought He had the whole world in His hands." You could tell I was highly influenced by Perry Como.

The good sister then explained to me the facts of shoulders, which is about as close to the facts of life as she ever got (or was permitted at that school). Shoulders, she said, are the most mobile joints of the entire body. (Which is why it's so easy to dislocate them.) They were created to help man throw a football, carry the groceries for Mom, and make the sign of the cross.

Shoulders are not related to the ears in any way, other than the fact that they are below them. You do not need to hunch forward and place your shoulders closer to the television set in order to hear better.

Shoulders do not hang low and are not supposed to wobble to and fro.

Strong shoulder and chest muscles are a must when it comes to lifting, pushing, and pulling, as well as carrying heavy loads and shutting the closet door when you have too much junk stuffed in there. There is a great tendency for shoulders to stoop as people get older, which is not so much a sign of old age as weak muscles and lack of exercise. (So shame on you if you look like the Hunchback of Notre Dame!)

The shoulder muscles work with the chest, neck, back, and arms, so the entire torso works together in harmony. (Just hum a few bars . . .)

The shoulder area is referred to by body professionals as the shoulder girdle. I mention this only because girdles are something we all relate to so well. The girdle consists of the scapula, or shoulder blade, and the clavicle, or collarbone. A ball and socket joint gives the maximum when it comes to movement and has just about unlimited range because of its structure. Exactly how strong that joint is in each person depends on how developed the muscles are in that area.

While I have yet to have any student come to one of my classes and complain about fat shoulders, it is essential to exercise the shoulders because of their relationship to the neck, chest, and arms.

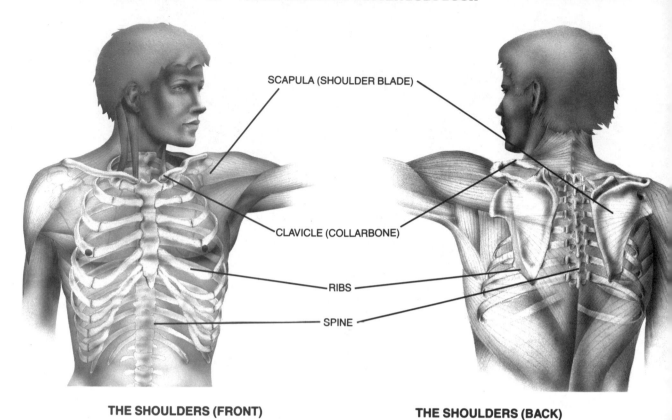

THE SHOULDERS (FRONT)

THE SHOULDERS (BACK)

Shoulder Moulders

1. "Shoulder Boy," a famous song sung by the Shirelles when I was in high school.

2. Fritz Shoulder, famous Native American artist known for his bright-colored paintings of other Native Americans.

3. Tomb of the Unknown Shoulder, commemorative monument to the brave men who have fallen in battle.

4. "Put Your Head on My Shoulder," another high school fave.

5. SOFT SHOULDERS, highway sign indicating that the pavement alongside the highway will not support the weight of your car. (Has your car considered a sensible food plan?)

Tension and Your Shoulders

Want to show the world that you're stiff, uptight, angry, feeling rotten, riddled with tension, and having a problem dealing with anxiety? Here's how! Now, in one short, easy lesson, you can have the secret of the ages, the truth to looking like you have a real pain in the neck. Just adapt any of these simple symptoms to your body language:

- shoulders that are raised
- shoulders that are rounded
- shoulders that are lopsided.

How can you get your shoulders to distort without trying? Consider any of these trusty techniques:

- emotional problems
- bad work habits (hunching over a type-writer)
- carrying a handbag that's too big, too heavy, or on one side of the body (A briefcase can also cause this problem; so can carrying a heavy child.)
- bad breathing habits
- poor posture
- wearing shoulder pads in your sweat shirts that are too heavy
- carrying your ankle weights in your tote bag
- pregnancy aches and pains
- carrying a bamboo pole with water buckets on each end
- working full-time as a milkmaid
- even bad breath can make you stoop over.

The back of the neck and the tops of the shoulders are where more tension accumulates than in any other place in your body. (They must give good convention rates to all those tension cells.) Muscles become hard and tight, and this makes circulation more difficult and pain more frequent. The trick to ending the pain is to get the muscles relaxed and the blood flowing more smoothly. Remember: Tension comes from muscles that have not been used and that have become miserable because of inactivity. Tension bases are usually in areas of the body that don't get a normal workout in daily activity and must be exercised in a regular program in order to be put to proper use. Use it or lose it.

Shoulder Dos and Don'ts

To avoid creating problems with your shoulders and to help cure those you may already have:

- DO exercise your shoulders as part of your daily exercise plan.
- DON'T carry anything heavy (even your child) on one side of your body for a prolonged period of time.
- DO exercise your shoulders whenever they feel tense or tight. Shoulder exercises can be done in an office, while traveling, and in limited space, and you needn't be naked or in a leotard.
- DON'T squeeze the top of your neck to try to ease shoulder pain.
- DON'T hunch over your work, even for a short period of time.
- DO practice the best posture you've got and work to improve it.

SH1 Shoulder Shrugs

Position: standing, feet slightly apart.

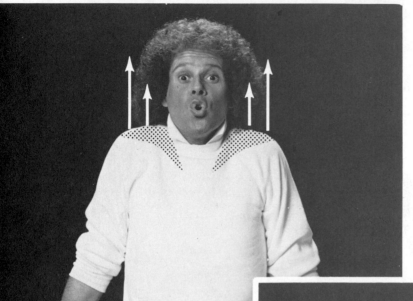

1. Lift your shoulders up to your ears while keeping your back straight.

2. Drop your shoulders down to their regular position.

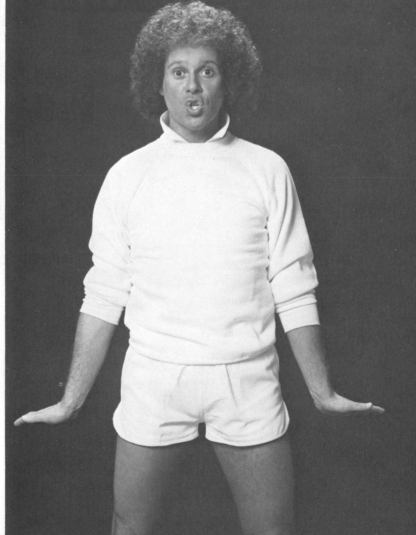

SH2 Forward and Backs

Position: standing, feet slightly apart.

1. Move your shoulders forward while keeping your back up and straight, then bring them back.

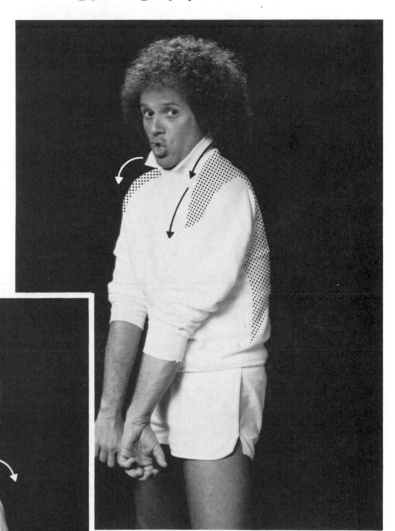

SH3 Shoulder Rounds

Position: standing, feet slightly apart.

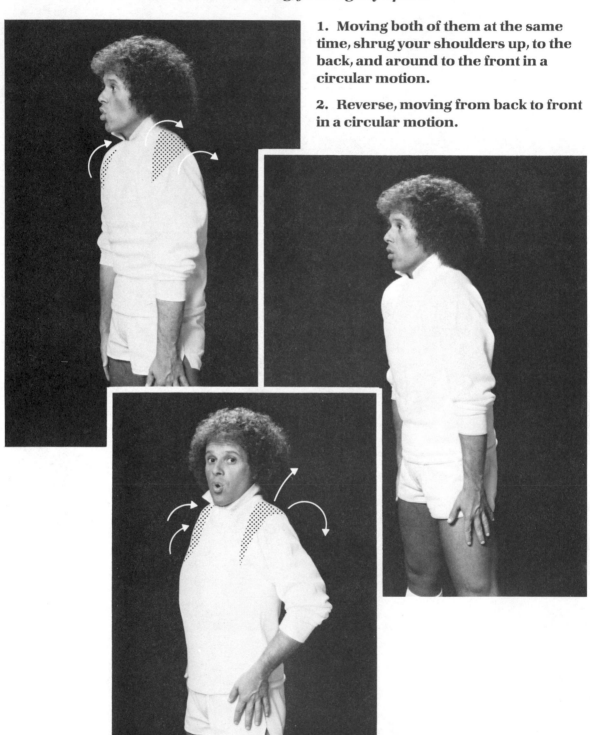

1. Moving both of them at the same time, shrug your shoulders up, to the back, and around to the front in a circular motion.

2. Reverse, moving from back to front in a circular motion.

SH4 Rowboats

Position: standing, feet slightly apart.

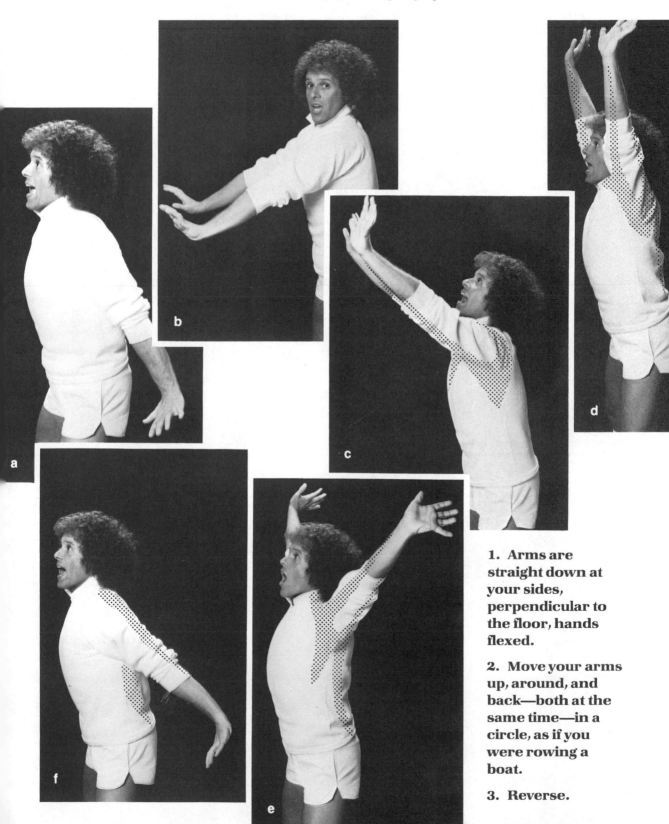

1. **Arms are straight down at your sides, perpendicular to the floor, hands flexed.**

2. **Move your arms up, around, and back—both at the same time—in a circle, as if you were rowing a boat.**

3. **Reverse.**

SH5 Elbow Pulls

Position: standing, feet slightly apart.

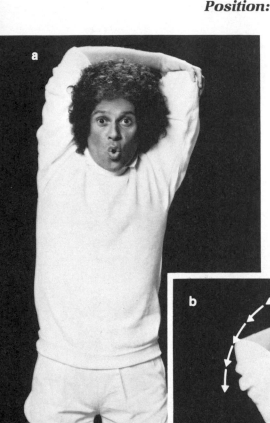

1. Raise both arms up over your head. Drop your right forearm to the left so that your elbow is pointing up.

2. With your right hand grab your left elbow.

3. Rest your left hand on your right elbow.

4. Pull down and to the right with your right hand.

5. Reverse.

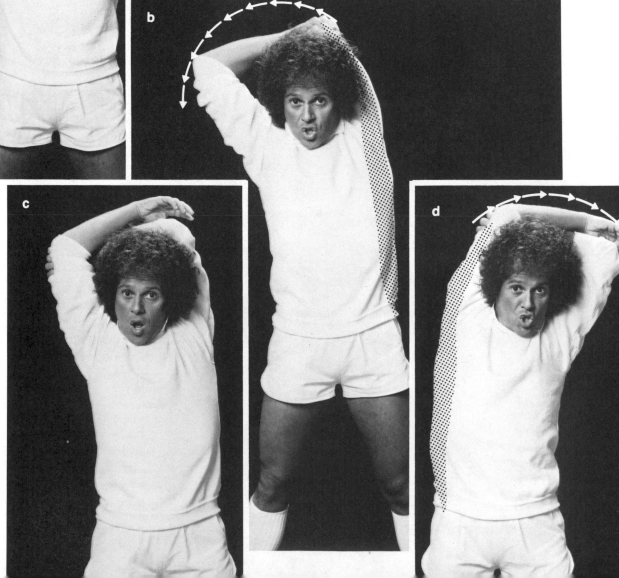

SH6 Shoulder Pyramids

Position: standing, feet apart, knees slightly bent.

1. Reach your arms out behind your back.

2. Grab one wrist with the opposite hand. (If you lace your fingers, the grasp may slip.)

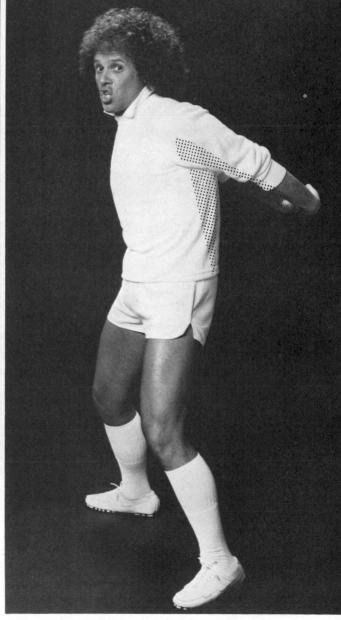

3. Pull back and up.

4. Reverse hands.

5. You should feel this in your upper back and your shoulder blades.

SH7 Shoulder Pyramids Forward

Position: standing, feet apart, knees slightly bent.

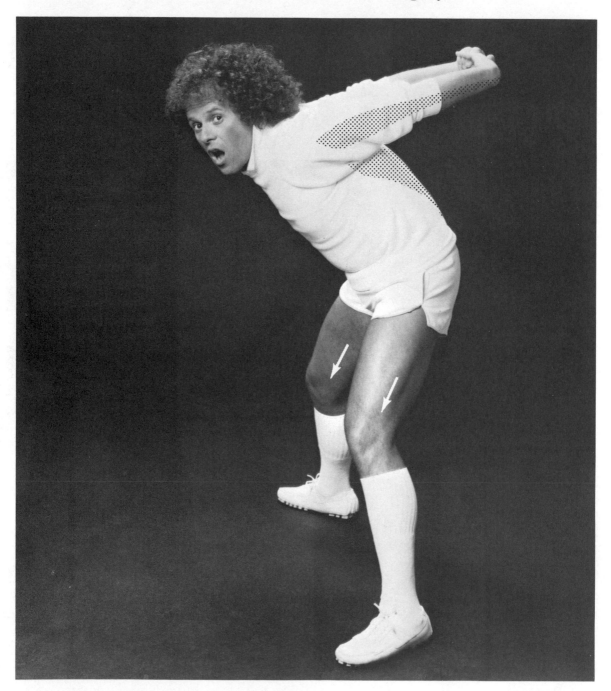

1. **Reach your arms out behind your back.**

2. **Grab one wrist with the opposite hand.**

3. **Pull back and up while bending forward.**

4. **Reverse hands.**

3

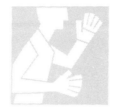

Arms and Hands

The Invention of Arms

We all know that arms have been considered extremely important throughout history. In fact, one of the reasons our forefathers fought the Revolutionary War was for the right to bear arms. And we all know that poor Venus de Milo would have been a totally more attractive woman if she just happened to have a set of arms. Arms have been vital to:

- the Supremes
- the Queen
- Michelangelo
- the Statue of Liberty
- Jesse James
- Armand Hammer
- Linda on *Sesame Street*.

Arms are made of three basic bones. The upper single bone is the humerus, which is built to bear and carry weight, while the two thinner bones, the ulna and the radius, extend the length of the limb and guide the hand.

The muscles in the arms were arranged by Noah so they come in twosies, or polite pairs. As one muscle contracts and shortens, the other relaxes and becomes longer. So when

*Boise.

you raise your arm in class to answer the teacher's question (What is the capital of Idaho?*), the biceps contracts and does the prime moving while the triceps relaxes. When you release your elbow and let your arm down, the reverse occurs. The way muscles work together is coordinated by the brain. You do not have a little foreman inside your body, shouting orders to those muscles—the adjustments you need are made automatically without conscious control. The muscles pull on the bones and make them do what your brain tells them to do.

When heavy loads are being carried, the weight of the arm, and its load, is transferred to the shoulder area—oops—the shoulder girdle, which is another example of why your entire body has to be in shape and why spot reducing is such a silly notion.

Your hands are made up of a series of small bones called the phalanges, which are themselves a series of bones. The fingers have no muscles, they are made up of tendons and ligaments, but the hand has lots of muscles, and they govern the action of the fingers. Exercise will not develop strength in your fingers, but it can produce stronger hands.

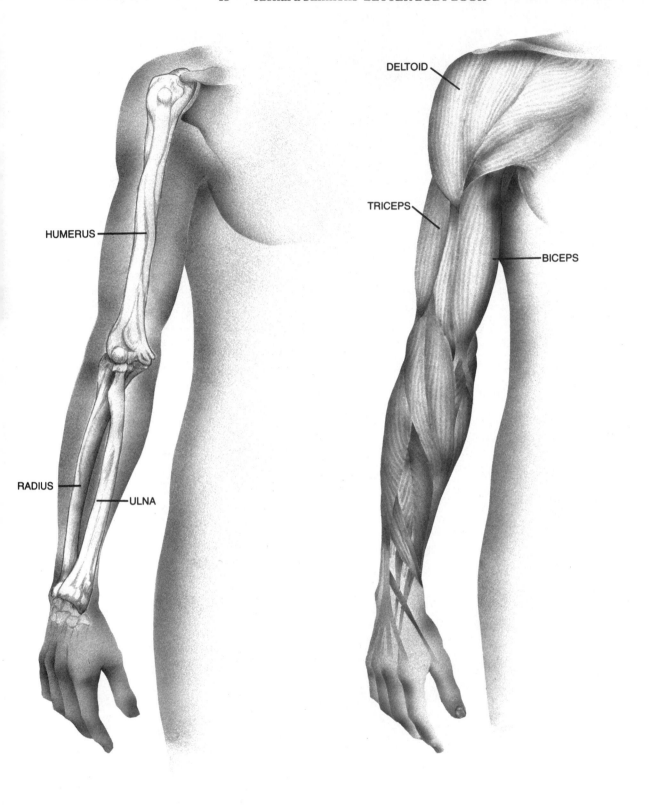

BONES OF THE ARM   **MUSCLES OF THE ARM**

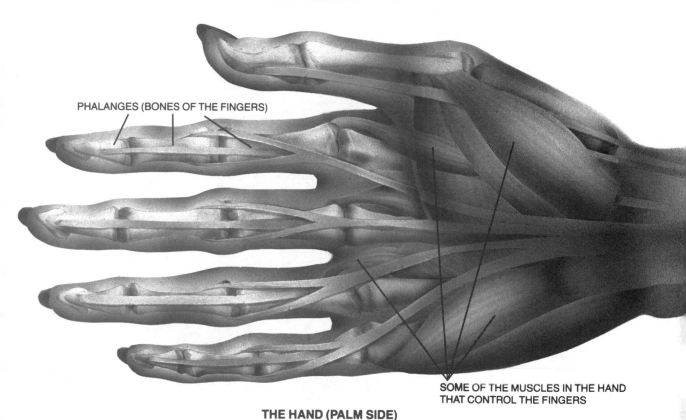

PHALANGES (BONES OF THE FINGERS)

SOME OF THE MUSCLES IN THE HAND
THAT CONTROL THE FINGERS

THE HAND (PALM SIDE)

Why does the gypsy woman want to read your palm? Because the hands happen to tell an awful lot about the human condition. You don't need to know a lifeline from a bloodline to be able to see the approach of disease or disaster. (You will meet a tall dark stranger.)

Doctor's pore over their patients' hands, checking the color and condition of fingernails, looking at the creases in the palms, testing flexibility, and studying the build of the thumbs—all as a way of finding disease.

Your Arm's Too Weak to Box with God

Tennis elbow is caused by repeated rotary forearm action with a strong handgrip. Massage and nonuse may ease the condition.

Rupture of the biceps can occur at any age but is most often seen in middle-aged people who are not in shape who suddenly try to lift or pull a heavy object that is beyond their capabilities.

Circulation problems: Since the hands and feet are the farthest away from the heart, they are the last parts of the body warmed and are the cause of pain or discomfort to many with circulation problems. Massage and exercise will often help circulation problems. Excessive smoking restricts the circulation, so if you are prone to cold hands and feet, you should stop smoking now. (You don't really smoke, do you? Shame on you.)

A1 Flex Fists

Position: standing, feet slightly apart.

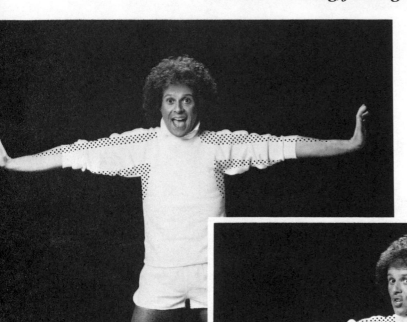

1. Arms are out to the side, parallel to the floor.

2. Flex your wrists so that your fingers are reaching for the sky.

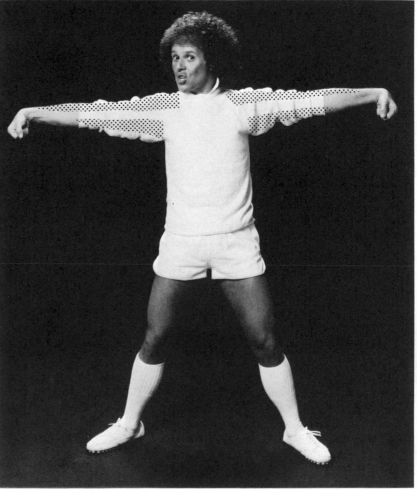

3. Curl your fingers into a fist as you flex and put your wrists down.

A2 Arm Circles

Position: standing, feet slightly apart.

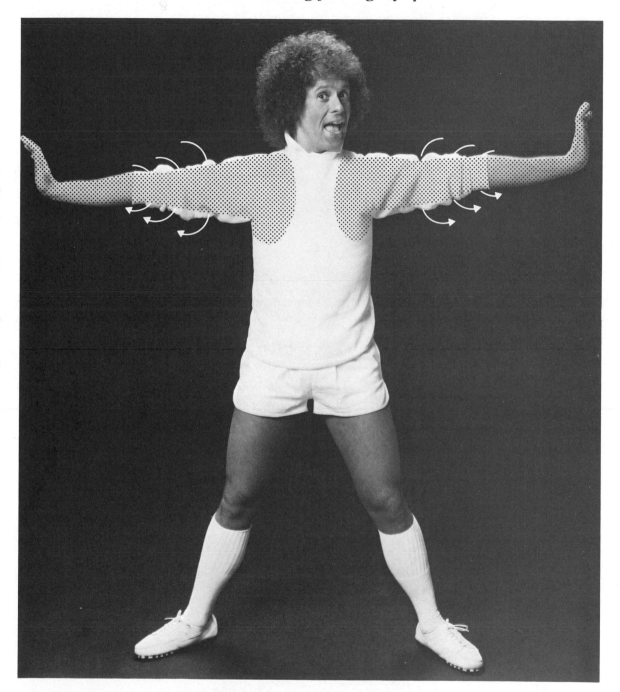

1. Arms are out to the side, parallel to the floor.

2. Flex your wrists so that your fingers point to the ceiling.

3. Circle your arms forward.

4. Reverse, circling your arms backward.

A3 Arm Circles—Flex Fist

Position: standing, feet slightly apart.

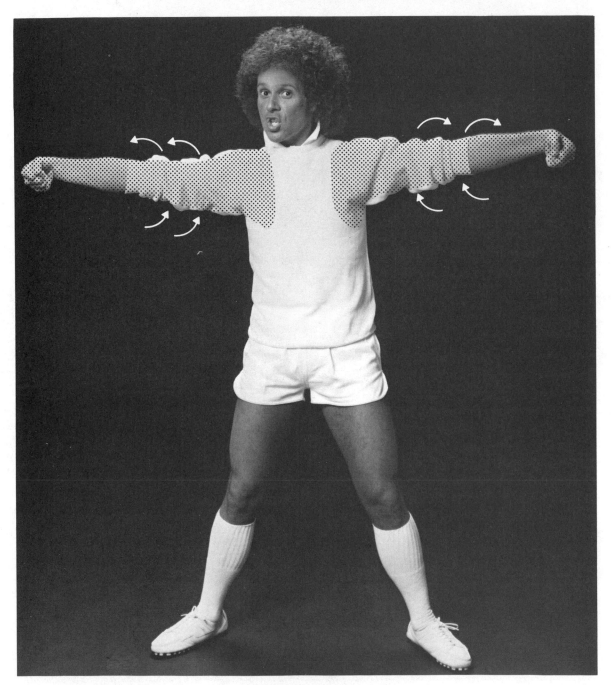

1. **Arms are out to the side, parallel to the floor.**

2. **Make fists and flex them up at the wrists.**

3. **Circle your arms forward.**

4. **Reverse, circling your arms backward.**

A4 Arm Twists

Position: standing, feet slightly apart.

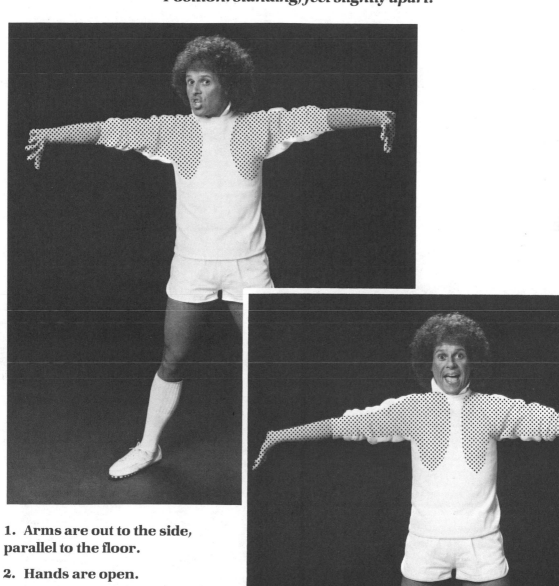

1. **Arms are out to the side, parallel to the floor.**

2. **Hands are open.**

3. **Twist your arms at the wrists, first forward, then back. This is the same kind of motion you use when you put salt on your food (which I know you don't do anymore).**

A5 Arm Pushes

Position: standing, feet slightly apart.

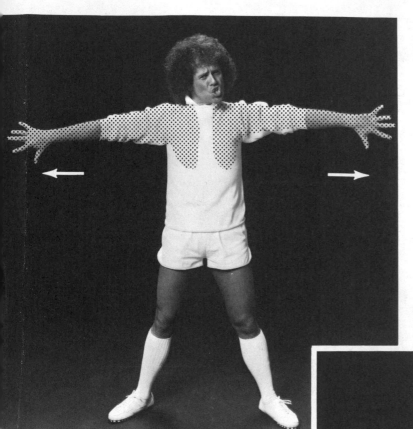

1. Arms are out to the side, parallel to the floor.

2. Hands are open.

3. Keep your shoulders straight and push your arms backward.

4. Reverse, pushing your arms forward.

5. You should also feel this in your back.

A6 Isometrics—Arms Out and Up

Position: standing, feet slightly apart.

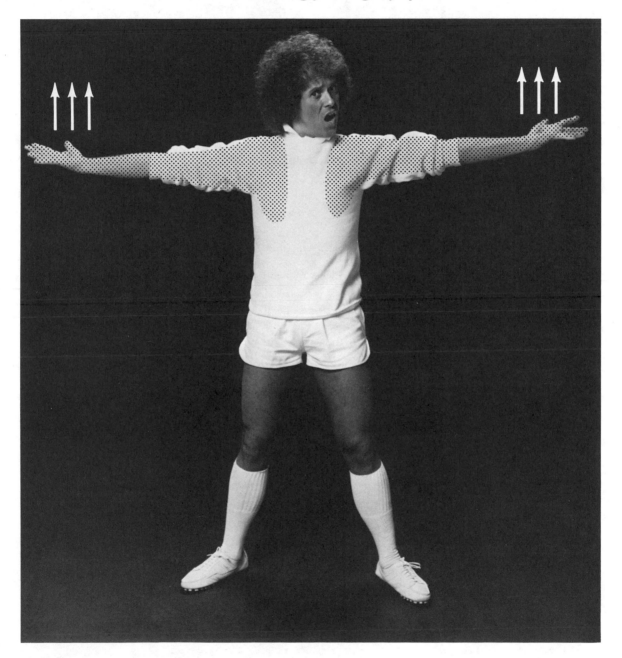

1. Arms are out to the side, parallel to the floor.

2. Palms are open, facing the ceiling.

3. Without bending your elbows pull your arms up, resisting the air.

A7 Isometrics—Arms Out and Down

Position: standing, feet slightly apart.

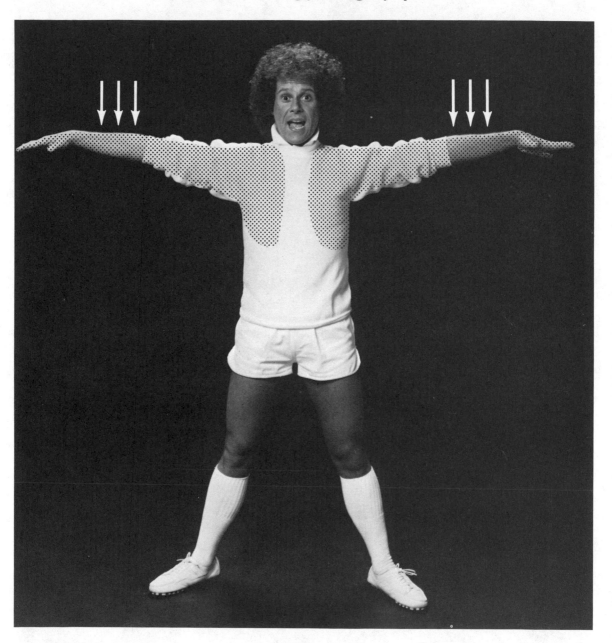

1. **Arms are out to the side, parallel to the floor.**

2. **Palms are open, facing the floor.**

3. **Without bending your elbows push your arms down, resisting the air.**

A8 Isometrics—Arms in Front

Position: standing, feet slightly apart.

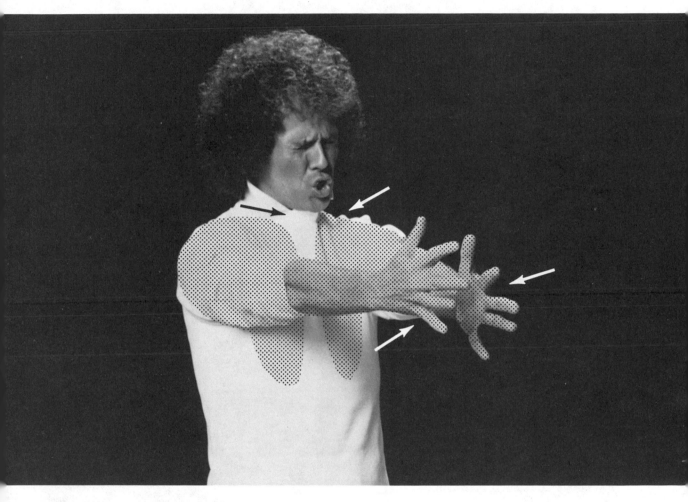

1. Reach your arms out in front of you.

2. Palms are facing each other.

3. Push in while resisting the air.

A9 Isometrics—Push Out

Position: standing, feet slightly apart.

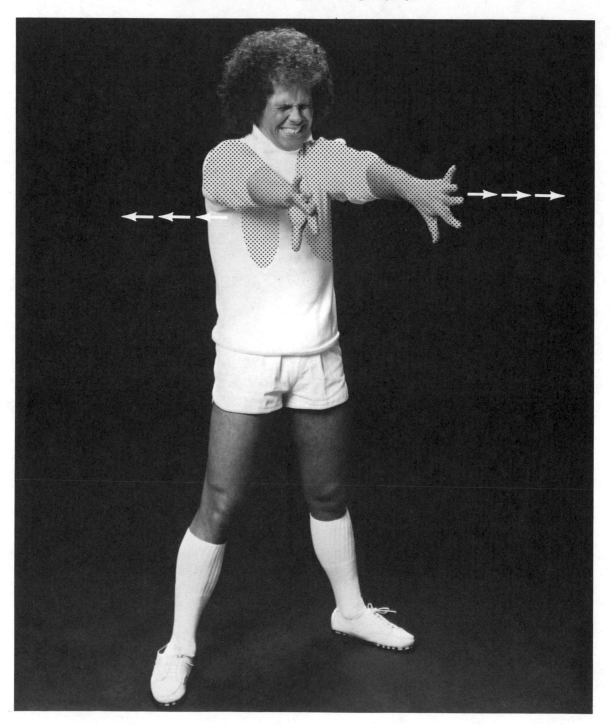

1. Reach your arms out in front of you.

2. Palms are facing away from each other.

3. Push out while resisting the air.

A10 Arm Hugs

Position: standing, feet slightly apart.

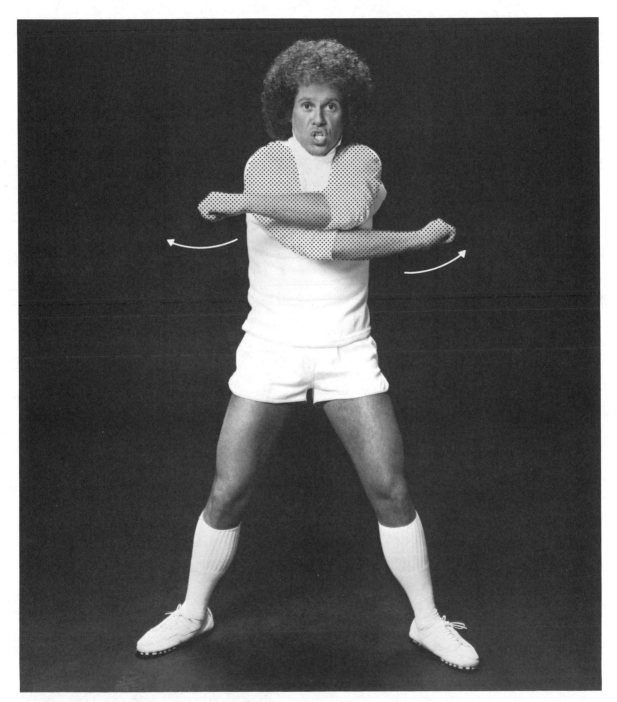

1. **Give yourself a hug, crossing your bent arms in front of you, with your hands in fists.**

2. **Change arms from front to back as you cross and uncross.**

3. **You should feel this in your upper back.**

A11 Straight Arm Hugs

Position: standing, feet slightly apart.

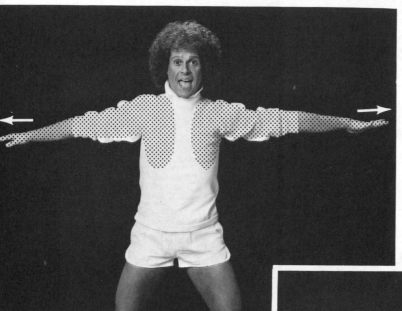

1. Arms are out to the side.

2. Cross your arms over your elbows in front of your body, right arm over left.

3. Reverse, with left arm crossing over right arm.

4. Keep your back straight.

5. Don't swing your arms.

6. You should feel this in your upper back.

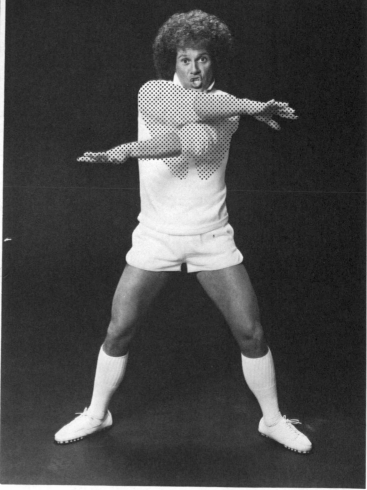

A12 Cross It Up—Palms Up

Position: standing, feet slightly apart, back straight.

1. Keep your arms straight out in front of you, palms up, and cross them left over right, right over left, until you are reaching above your head.

2. Cross at the elbows.

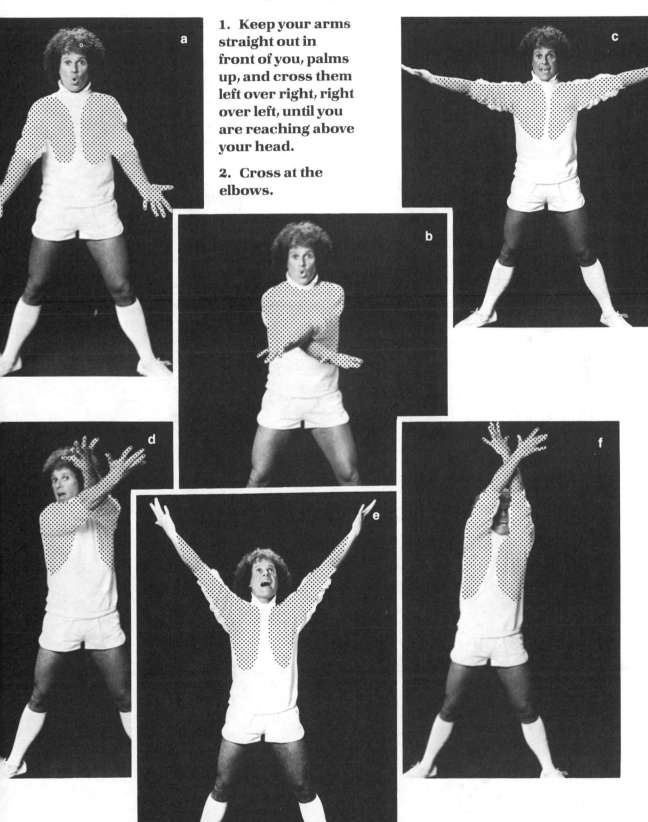

A13 Cross It Up—Palms Down

Position: standing, feet slightly apart, back straight.

1. Keep your arms straight out in front of you, palms down, and cross them left over right, right over left, until you are reaching above your head.

2. Cross at the elbows.

3. You should feel this in your back.

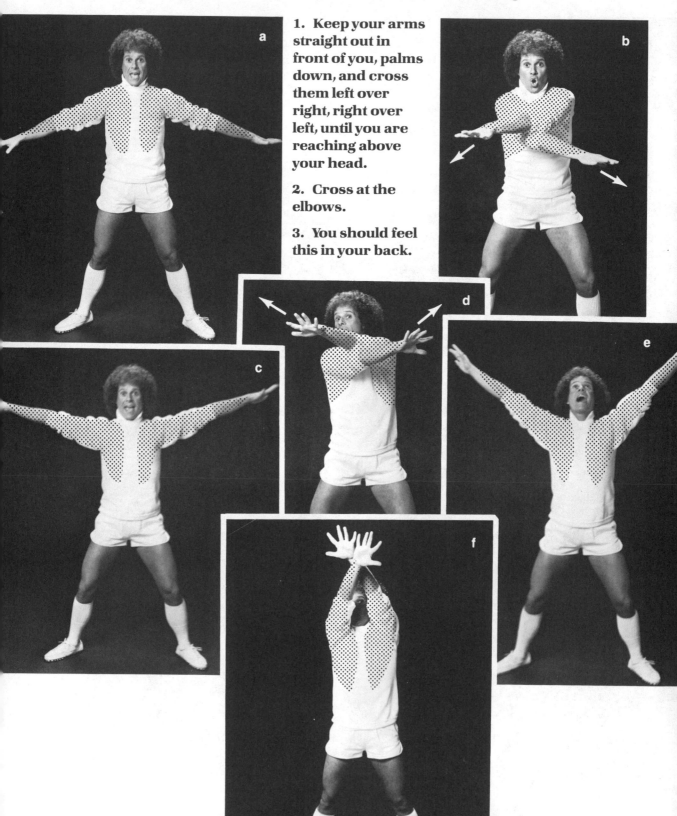

A14 Flex and Points

Position: standing, feet slightly apart.

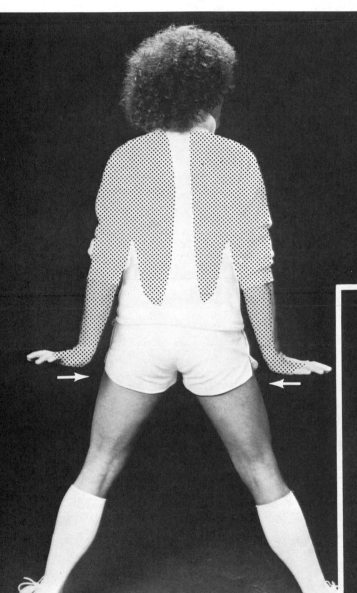

1. Arms arc down to the side, hands are flexed up at the wrist.

2. Keeping hands flexed, bring arms behind your back, trying to meet your wrists behind you.

3. Point hands, fingers toward each other, flex hands with fingers away, point hands, flex hands, etc.

4. Keep shoulders back and chest up.

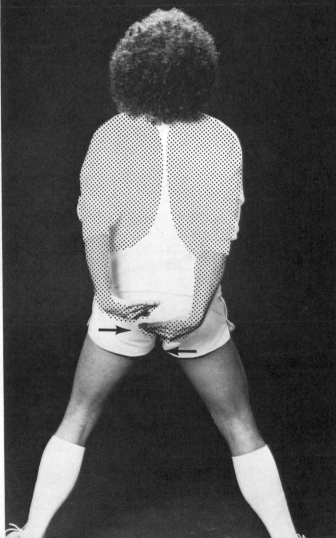

A15 Arm Crosses in Back

Position: standing, feet slightly apart.

1. Cross arms behind you, left over right, right over left.

2. Keep palms open.

3. Keep elbows straight.

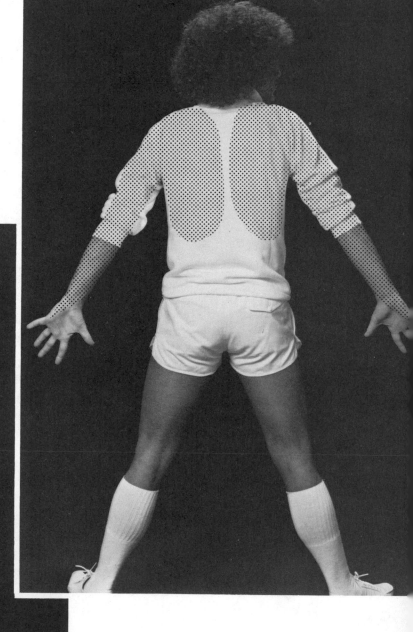

A16 Arm Lifts to the Back

Position: standing, feet slightly apart, knees slightly bent.

1. Keep shoulders back. Arms are at your sides with hands flexed.

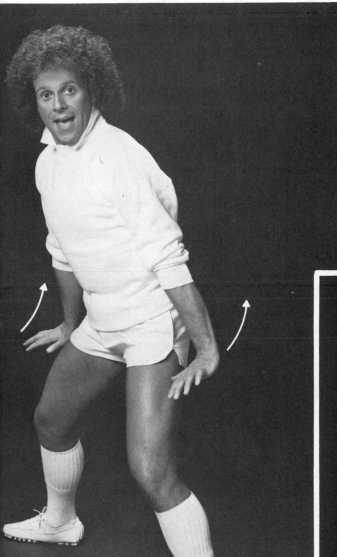

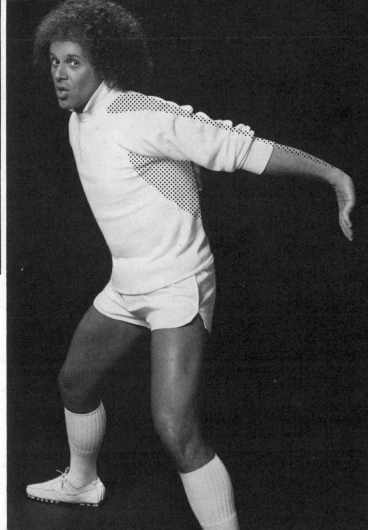

2. Bring arms straight back and lift without swinging.

A17 Armpit Power

Position: standing, feet slightly apart.

1. **Arms are down at sides, hands in fists.**

2. **Bend at the elbows with arms in front at shoulder level.**

3. **Open arms out so that they are straight.**

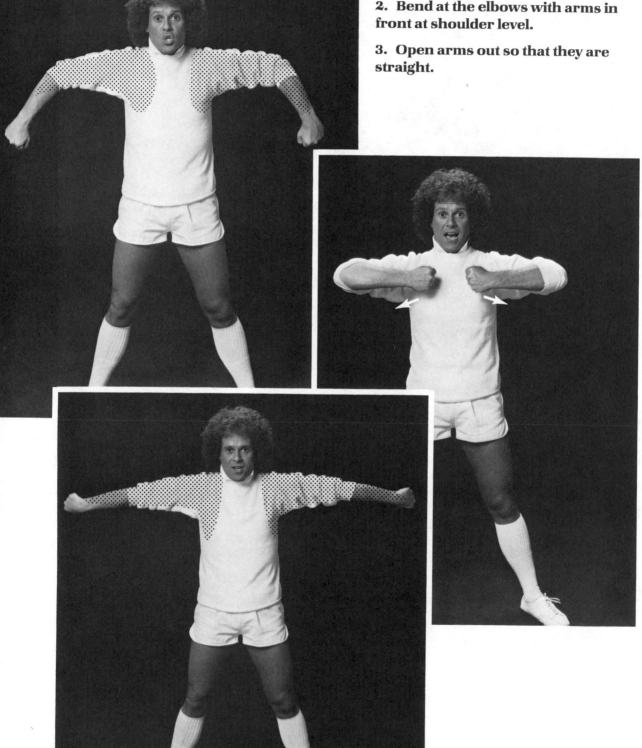

A18 Diagonal Arm Stretches

Position: standing, feet slightly apart.

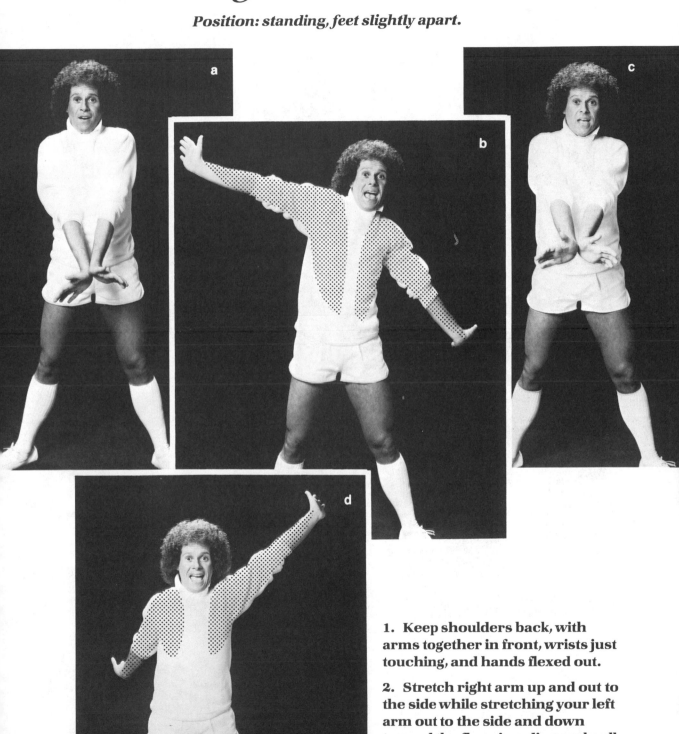

1. **Keep shoulders back, with arms together in front, wrists just touching, and hands flexed out.**

2. **Stretch right arm up and out to the side while stretching your left arm out to the side and down toward the floor in a diagonal pull.**

3. **Return from the stretch by letting wrists meet in front of you.**

4. **Alternate sides.**

A19 Hands, Fingers, and Wrists

Position: standing, feet slightly apart.

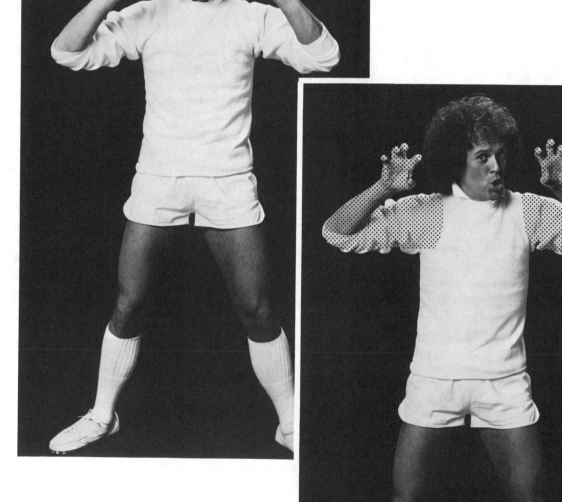

1. Hold hands up, elbows relaxed.

2. Claw an imaginary ball.

3. Release claw position, claw, release, etc.

A20 Spiderwebs

Position: standing, feet slightly apart.

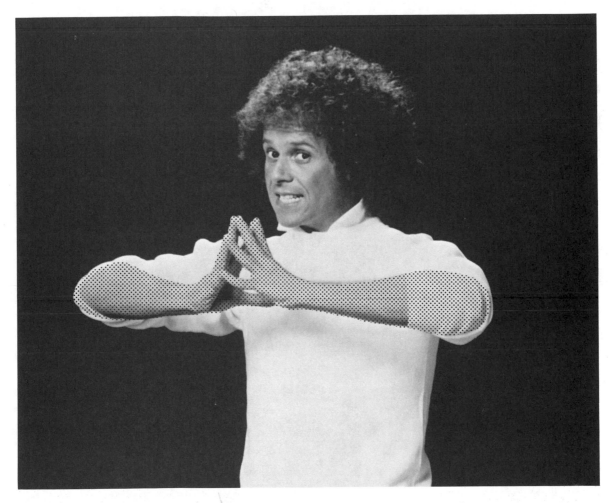

1. Keeping shoulders back and back straight, press fingers together to form a "church steeple" like when you were a kid.

2. Press each finger against its opposite finger.

A21 Finger Rolls

Position: standing, feet slightly apart.

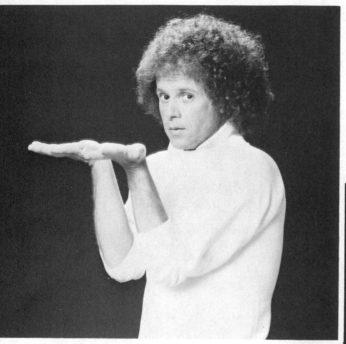

1. Arms are held out in front of you, elbows bent, with the palms open.

2. Roll fingers into the palms, roll them out, in, out, etc.

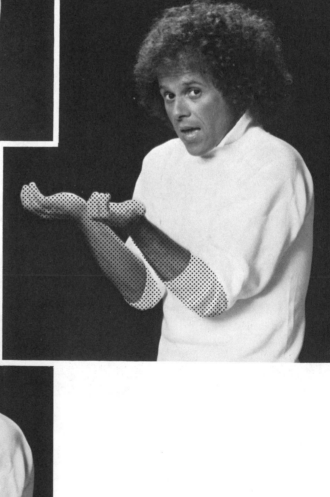

A22 *Wrist Rotations*

Position: standing, feet slightly apart.

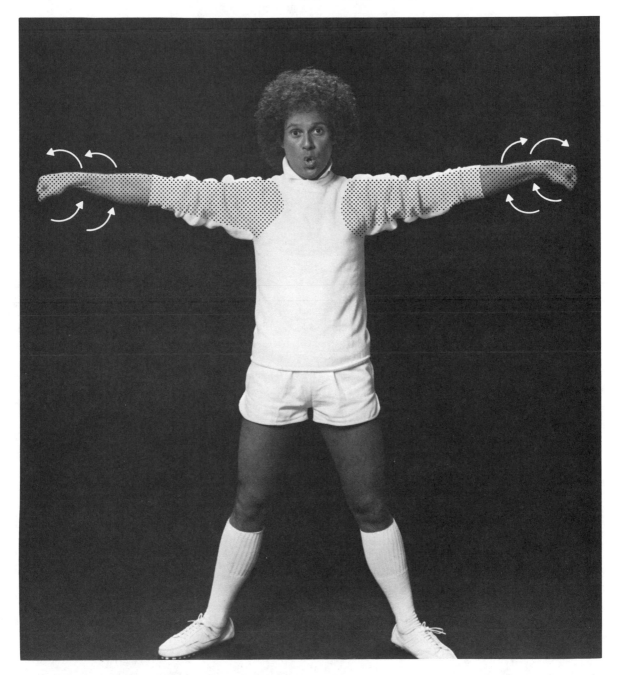

1. Arms are held straight out to the side.

2. Make fists and rotate them in a circle forward, then backward. Roll that wrist, c'mon and roll wrist roll.

4

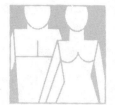

His and Her Chest

The Torso, of Course-O

The area between the shoulders and the hips (real men don't have waists) is called the torso. It is probably derived from the Spanish word *torro,* for "bull," because this is the area where a guy can look stocky faster than anywhere else. The male and female torsos are radically different. (I'm not trying to be sexist folks, but facts is facts.) BUT the inside skeletons are more or less the same. Just note that the male pelvic girdle is narrower than the female's (for obvious reasons), which is why men don't have waists and women do.

The torso includes the area known as the rib cage, with its twelve ribs. The first seven ribs are attached by cartilage directly to the sternum, or breastplate, in the front of your body and protect the heart. Each of the next three ribs is attached by cartilage to the rib above it. The eleventh and twelfth ribs do not attach and are therefore called floating ribs, which are hard to find. If you want to count your ribs someday, start at the top of your collarbone, which is on top of rib number two. (This is an activity that is especially fun if you are [A] bored in class, [B] bored at a cocktail party, or [C] lacking in conversation on a first date.) If you aren't too overweight, you should be able to touch about seven ribs.

WARNING TO FIRST DATERS: It's harder to find the ribs in a female than in a male, but you can have fun trying.

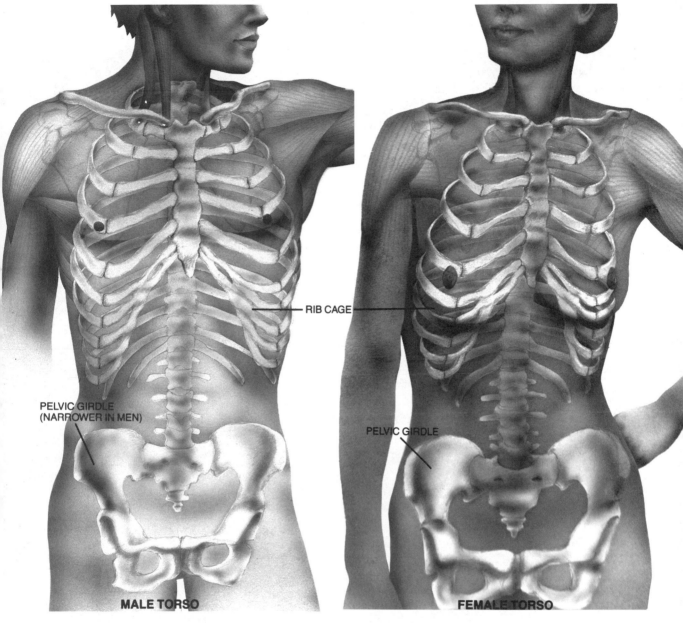

RIB CAGE

PELVIC GIRDLE
(NARROWER IN MEN)

PELVIC GIRDLE

MALE TORSO

FEMALE TORSO

Chest Nuts

The chest protects the heart and lungs and houses the diaphragm, and then gives way to the liver and the stomach, where the ribs are no longer attached in the front of the bod. Because of the bones in the chest, there's less opportunity to get fat where the ribs are. Once you get away from the confines of the skeleton, it's very, very easy to get fat, which is why so many people have ripples and love handles, and tires or circles of fatty deposits.

Fat just loves to build up between the interior organs and the hips, because there is more room for those little suckers (fat cells) to get in there than in any other part of the body.

The best way to keep this fat out is to (A) hire a guard to fit inside your body and say scram every time a fat cell comes looking for property or (B) exercise regularly so you have a firm body structure and less room for squatters.

Bosom Buddies

Every woman in the world seems to worry about the size of her breasts. They're either too big or too small. But, ladies, can we talk seriously for a minute? It's not how big they are, it's how FIRM they are. Now, put that in your Maidenform and smoke it.

Exercise cannot make your breasts larger or smaller. Exercise can strengthen the muscles that support the breasts, which will make them look tremendously better. Pregnancy, nursing, jogging, and bad posture all help create sagging breasts. Exercise prevents the big droop. And, as an added bonus, you'll find that the chest muscles are so related to the shoulders and arms that the same exercises that improve your bust also help keep your upper arms from becoming flabby.

For better boosies you need to get to work on your pecs (yes, women have pecs, too), as well as the serratus, the deltoid, the latissimus dorsi, the biceps, and the triceps muscles. You don't need to work out with weights or fancy machines, and you don't need bust-developing ointments. You just need determination.

Also remember that as you lose weight your breasts will reduce as well. If the muscles aren't worked on, your new figure will have some sorry-looking trophies. Sure, you can have surgery to give you an uplift, but exercise will hold up the good doctor's works of arts. Without exercise you'll be needing more surgery in less than five years!

Breast size is mostly genetic, and while weight gain and pregnancy will affect your bustline, only exercise can keep you trim.

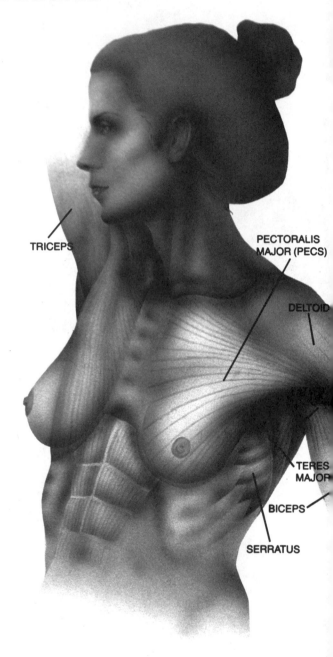

TRICEPS

PECTORALIS MAJOR (PECS)

DELTOID

TERES MAJOR

BICEPS

SERRATUS

MUSCULATURE OF THE FEMALE CHEST

C1 Push-Ups—Regular

Position: on mat, in traditional push-up position.

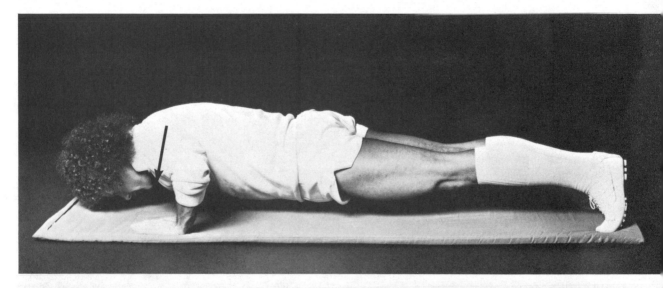

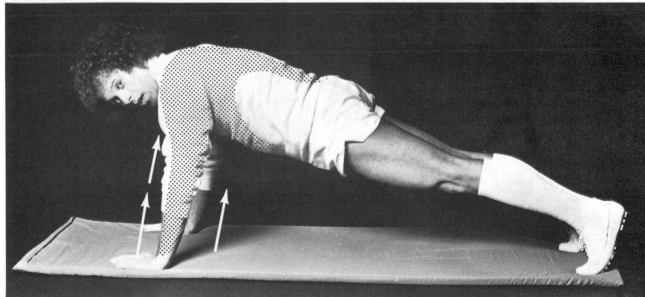

1. Palms are out in front of you, fingers facing forward.

2. You should be balancing on your toes.

3. Push your body weight up and down as you raise and lower yourself by bending only your elbows. Don't get swayback doing this, please.

C2 *Push-Ups—Hands Out*

Position: on mat, in traditional push-up position.

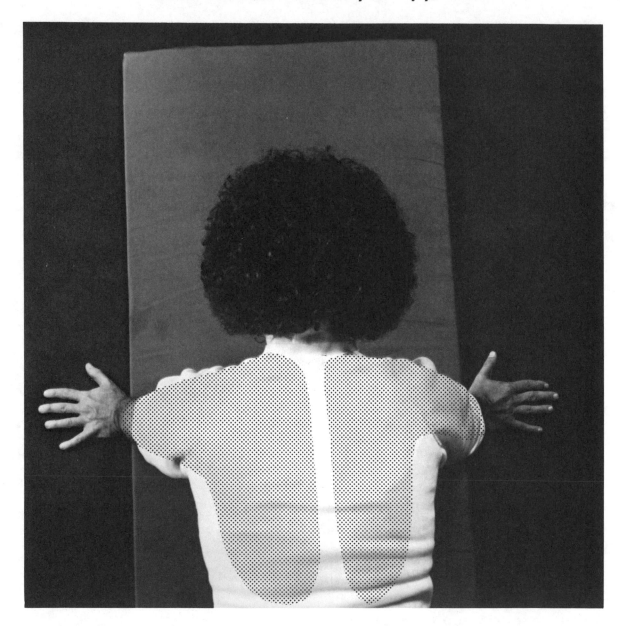

1. Your hands should be facing out, fingers pointing at opposite walls.

2. Raise and lower yourself by bending only at your elbows.

C3 Push-Ups—Hands In

Position: on mat, in traditional push-up position.

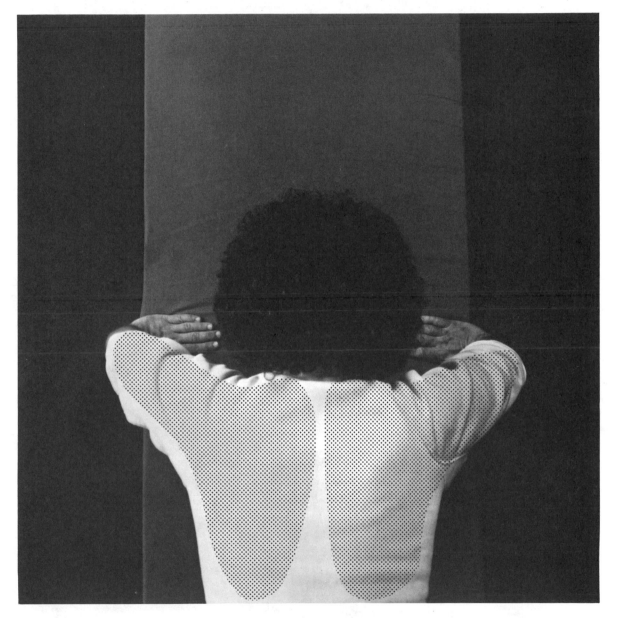

1. **Your hands should be facing in toward your body.**

2. **Raise and lower yourself by bending only at your elbows.**

C4 Elbow Pushes

Position: standing, feet slightly apart, shoulders back.

1. Arms are held out in front of you.

2. Elbows are bent and parallel to each other, with palms facing the ceiling.

3. Wrists are apart, hands are flexed.

4. Press elbows together.

5. Release.

6. You should feel this in your chest.

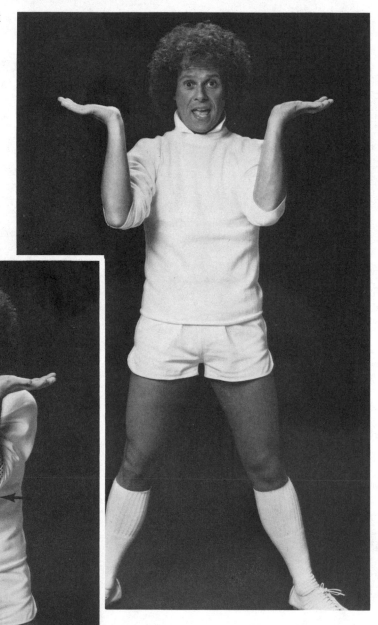

C5 Chest—Her
Palm Pushes

Position: standing, feet slightly apart, shoulders back.

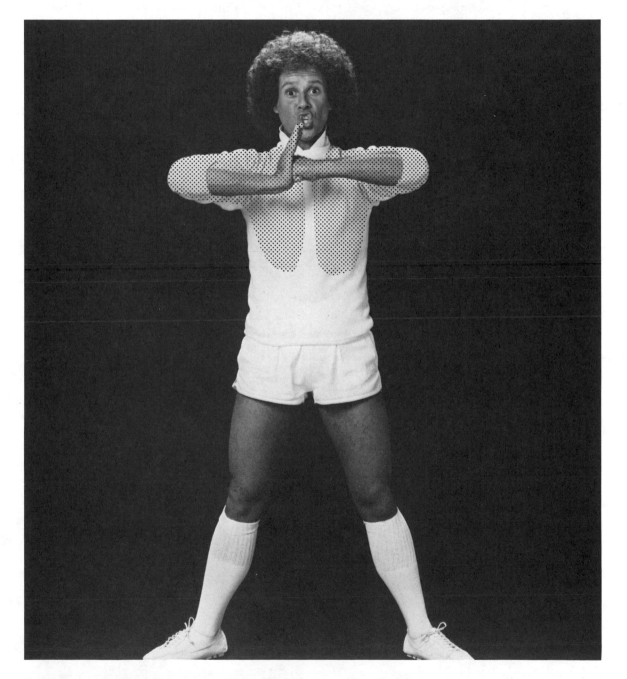

1. Arms are out in front, parallel to the floor, with elbows bent.

2. Press your left fist into your right palm. Then press your right fist into your left palm.

C6 *Prayer Pushes*

Position: standing, feet slightly apart, shoulders back.

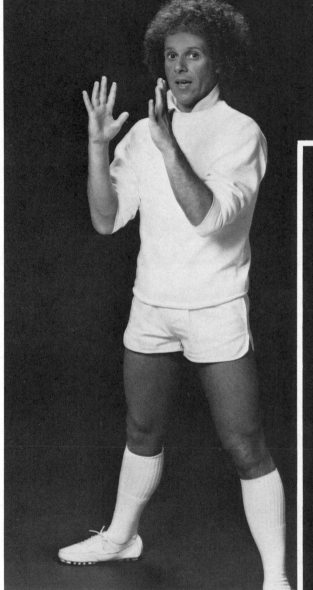

1. With arms out in front of you, elbows bent, place elbows and wrists together.

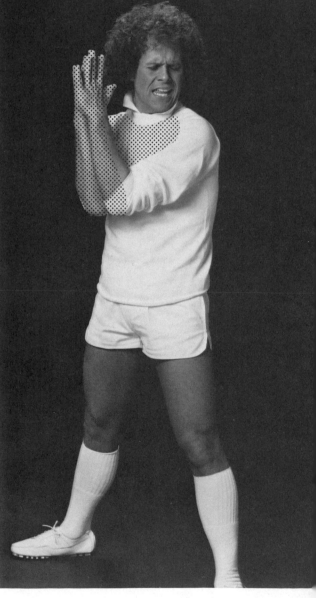

2. Press your palms together as if you were praying.

3. Press, release, press, release, etc.

C7 Backward Push-Ups

Position: sitting on mat with your body in a straight line.

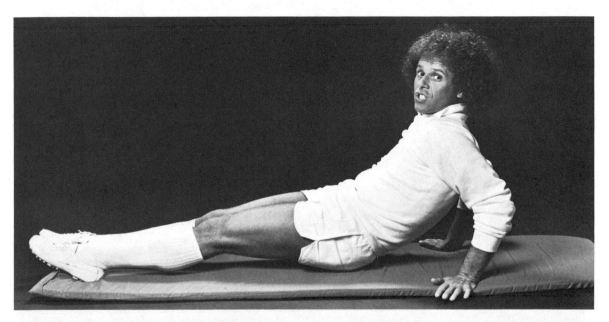

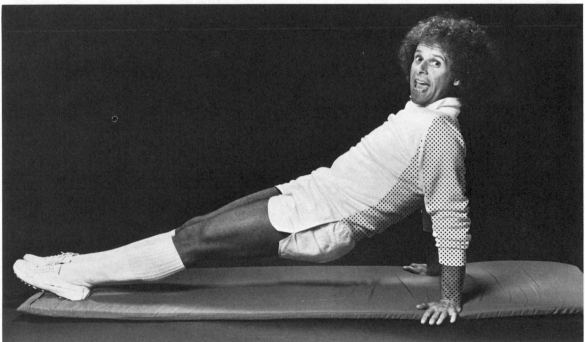

1. Put your hands on the mat behind you, fingers facing out. Raise your body up and down doing a backward push-up. (Get a look at the name, kids.)

2. This is not a pelvic tilt. Your elbows do all the moving, not your bottom. Keep your rear end off the ground at all times.

3. You should feel this in your whole back.

C8 Forward Push-Ups with Bent Knees

Position: on mat, in traditional push-up position.

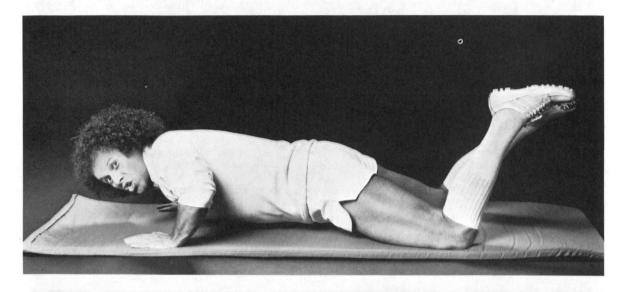

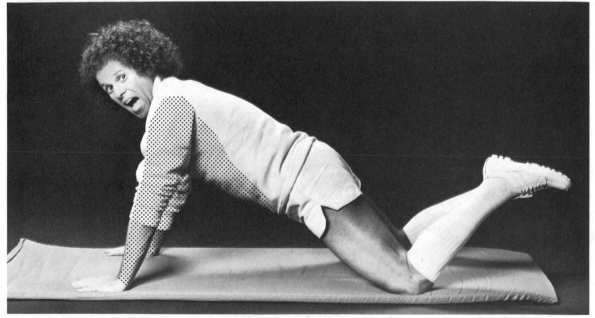

1. Your body should be in a straight line.

2. Bend your knees, keeping your feet off the ground.

3. Raise and lower yourself by bending your elbows.

C9 Backward Push-Ups with Bent Knees

Position: sitting on mat, with your body in a straight line.

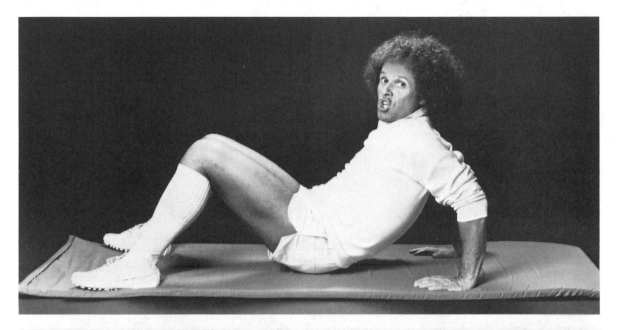

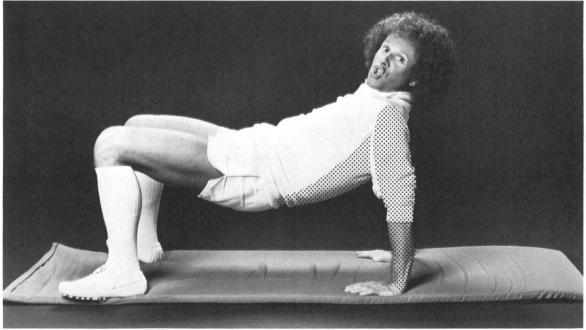

1. Put your hands on the mat behind you and bend your knees, with your feet flat on mat.

2. Raise and lower yourself, using your elbows only.

5

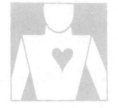

Heart

Heartlands

Regular exercise is one of the nicest things you can give your heart—Valentine's Day or no. Your heart is muscle, and you are greatly responsible for the shape and tone of that muscle. As the heart walls strengthen through exercise the heart pumps blood more efficiently and circulation improves. Thus the other muscles in your body can work better and harder, because more oxygen is reaching them. When more oxygen gets in, a person feels better and has more energy. Everyone who wants more energy, throw this book up in the air and shout "HURRAY!"

Aerobic exercise is the kind that takes extra air into the lungs and is therefore the best for the heart. (Of course, you need other types of exercise for others parts of your body. Aerobic exercise does not necessarily help you lose weight.)

Good aerobic exercises include: brisk walking, jogging, swimming, cycling, jumping rope, cross-country skiing, canoeing, and any specially designed aerobic exercise or dance class.

The fit heart works very efficiently and can pump more slowly because it is so strong. The unfit heart—the ca-ca heart, as they call it in nonmedical terms—has weak pumping action, so it has to go lub-dub more and more frequently.

Let Me Call You Sweet Heart

The adult heart does not look the way Cupid told you it would. In fact, when I found out what hearts REALLY looked like, I walked right out of class and into the men's room. Yuck. But I guess it's part of growing up. So, if any of you didn't know that Cupid was a liar, here's the honest to goodness truth. A human heart really looks like this:

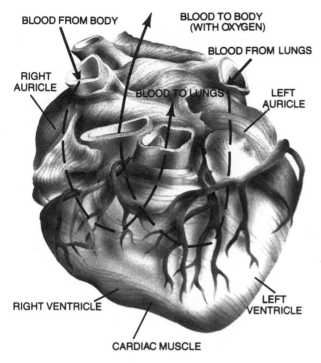

BLOOD FROM BODY

BLOOD TO BODY
(WITH OXYGEN)

BLOOD FROM LUNGS

RIGHT
AURICLE

BLOOD TO LUNGS

LEFT
AURICLE

RIGHT VENTRICLE

LEFT
VENTRICLE

CARDIAC MUSCLE

**THE HUMAN HEART
(SEEN FROM THE FRONT)**

It's not heart-shaped, at all; it's more pear-shaped and is about the size of your fist. When you pledge allegiance to the flag, you can feel it lub-dubbing in your chest, safely cradled behind a whole bunch of ribs.

The heart has four chambers—kind of like one of those movie theaters in a shopping mall where they're showing four different features at the same time—and they work in teams, just like at camp. The right side of the heart gets the blood that has passed through the vessels and sends it to the lungs. In the lungs the blood gives up the carbon dioxide and gets oxygen. The left side of the heart receives the newly oxygenated blood from the lungs and sends it throughout your whole body on the Chattanooga Choo Choo.

The wall of the heart is made of cardiac muscle, and the action of this muscle pumps the blood to its destination. Heavy exercise (that means more than getting out of bed or turning on the television set) increases the stroke volume of the heart so that the heart is able to pump the same amount of blood throughout the body with fewer beats. This is good for the home team.

Over one million people in the United States alone die of heart disease each year. Another one million will live through a heart trauma. (And I don't mean that no one will send them a valentine.) Better nutrition and the right kind of exercise can lower these statistics.

Heartening News

One of the most frequently asked questions I answer is, "Should I exercise before or after I eat?"

No, this is not a stomach question, this is really a heart question. Here's why: When you exercise, your heart pumps faster, doing a little extra work. After you eat, blood goes to your stomach to aid the digestive process. If you try exercising while all the blood is in your stomach, your poor little heart has to work not double time, but quadruple time—that's four times as hard. And that is just too great a strain for a normal person to bear.

Here are the rules: Exercise BEFORE you eat so that the blood is not in your stomach. If you eat a light meal, wait at least one and a half hours before exercising. (I know you only eat light meals.) If you eat a heavy meal, wait at least two hours. Walking after a meal is okay and actually helps digestion. Sleeping after a meal is rotten and actually helps you get fat.

YES, YOU CAN EXERCISE ON AN EMPTY STOMACH. (It's even a good idea.) Remember: Exercising after eating is bad for your heart.

Up in Smoke

I'm not going to give you a big lecture about smoking. I just want you to remember a few simple things:

• A person who smokes a pack of cigarettes a day has three times the chance of dying (yes, I said dying) from a heart attack.

• Cigarette smoking produces carbon monoxide. Now, you know that if you want to commit suicide, you can go into the garage and turn on your car and choke on the fumes.

Smoking is committing suicide the slow way.

• The nicotine in cigarettes speeds up the heart rate, raises blood pressure, makes the blood more likely to clot, and also constricts the blood vessels. So your cloggy old blood can't get through your body anyway. Result? You die.

• I'm not even going to talk about the cancer stuff. After all, this is the chapter on hearts.

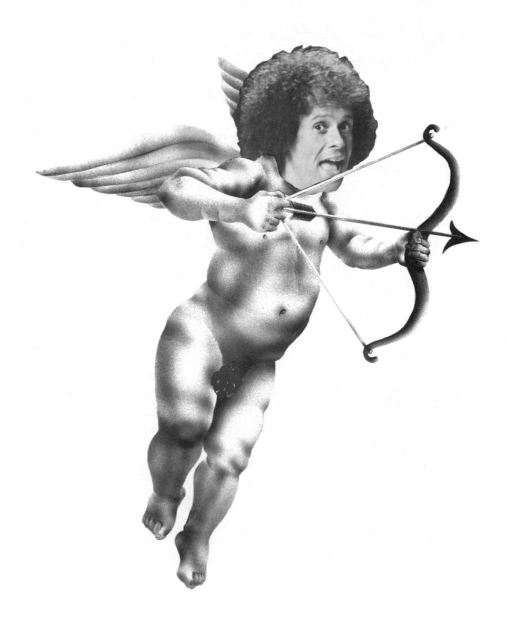

H1 Running in Place

Position: standing, shoulders back.

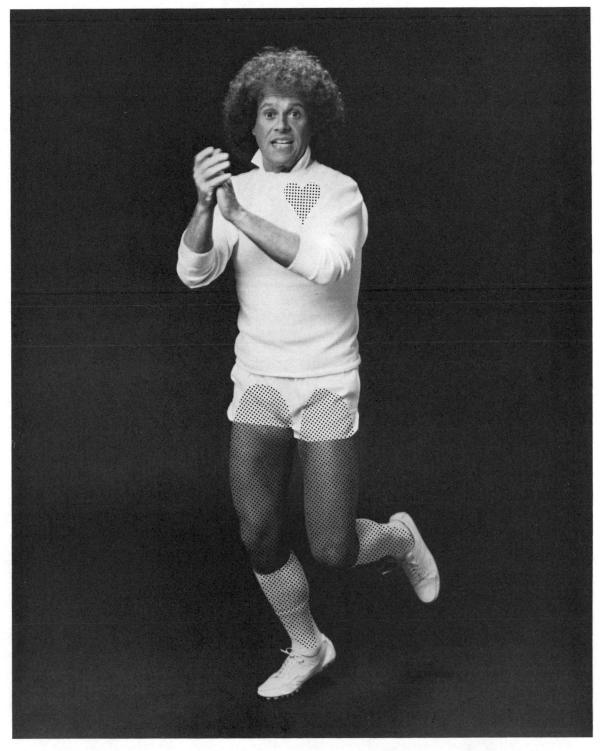

1. **Making sure that your heels touch the ground, run in place, 5–10 minutes.**

H2 Skippers *(I didn't say strippers. Don't get excited.)*

Position: standing, shoulders back.

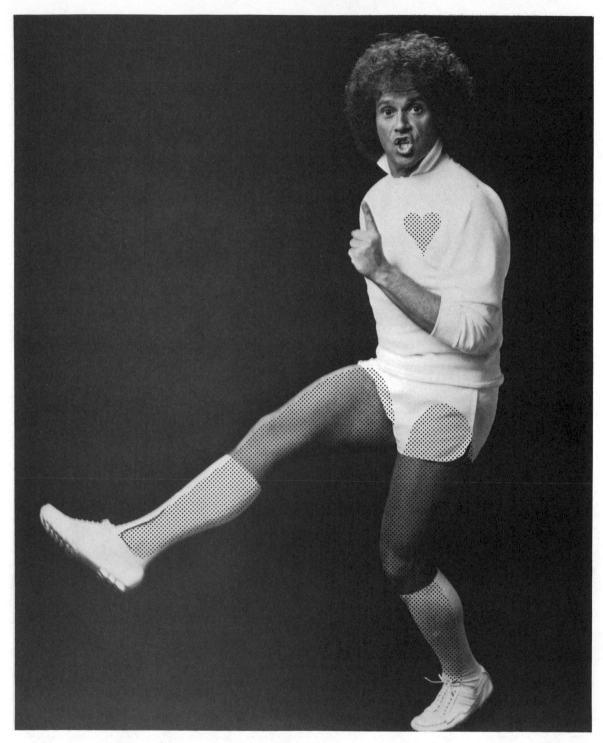

1. Skip your legs out in front of you without really going anywhere.

H3 Skips to the Side

Position: standing, shoulders back.

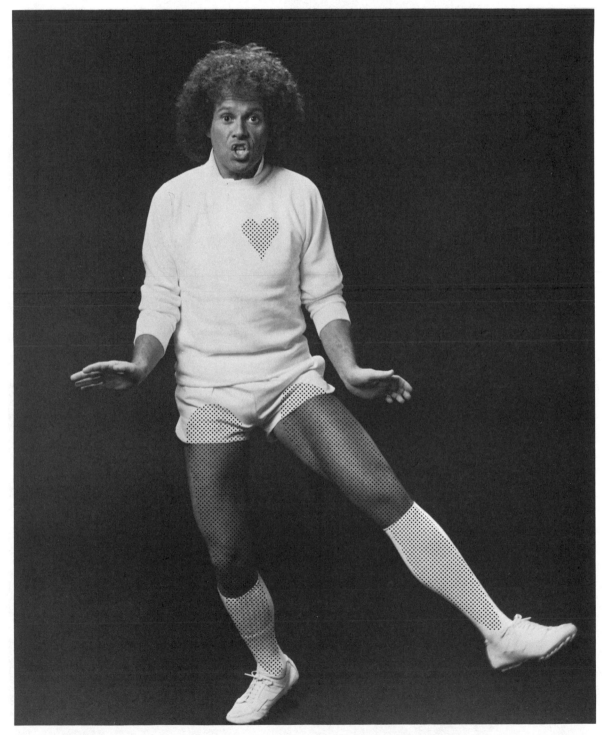

1. **While skipping, swing your right leg to the right, then your left leg to the left.**

2. **Alternate sides.**

H4 Twists and Jumps (Work It on Out)

Position: standing, shoulders back, feet together.

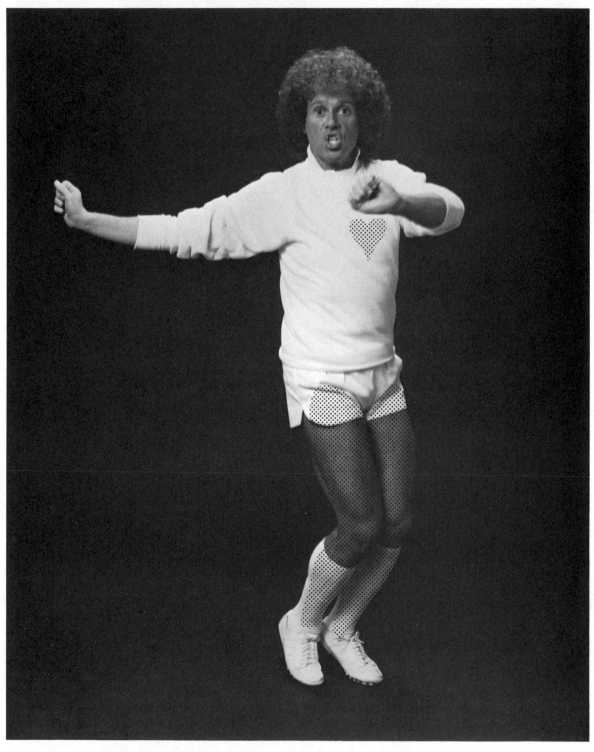

1. Twist from the waist from side to side, jumping as you twist.

H5 Open Twists

Position: standing, shoulders back, feet apart.

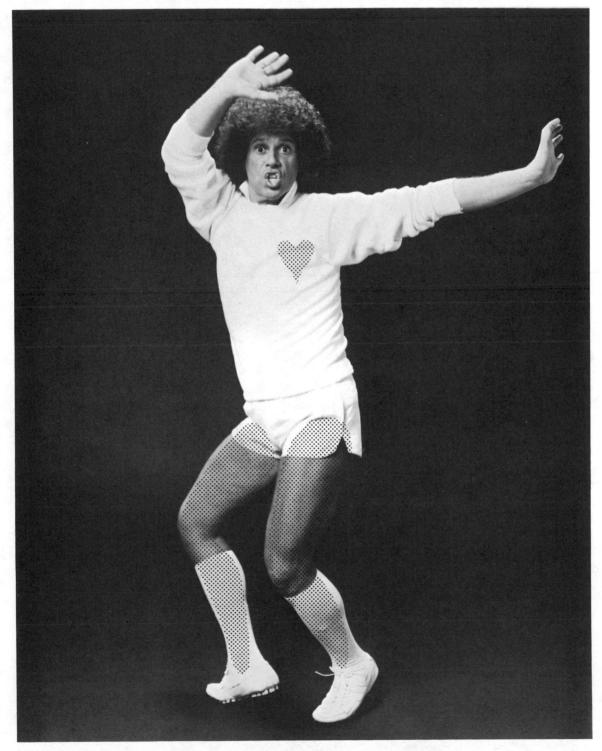

1. Twist from the waist from side to side, jumping as you twist.

H6 Side Kicks—Down

Position: standing, tummy in.

1. As your right leg kicks to the right side, your right arm goes down, with your fingers pointing down, and your left arm goes up.

2. As your left leg kicks to the left side, your left arm goes down, with your fingers pointing down, and your right arm goes up.

3. Alternate sides.

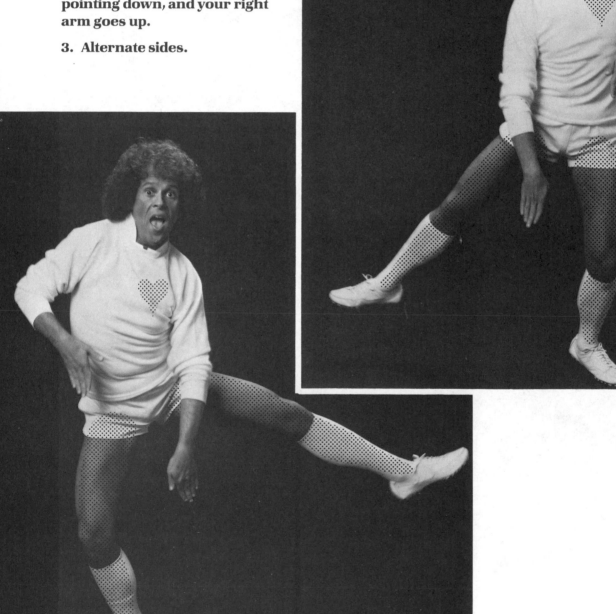

H7 Side Kicks—Up

Position: standing, tummy in.

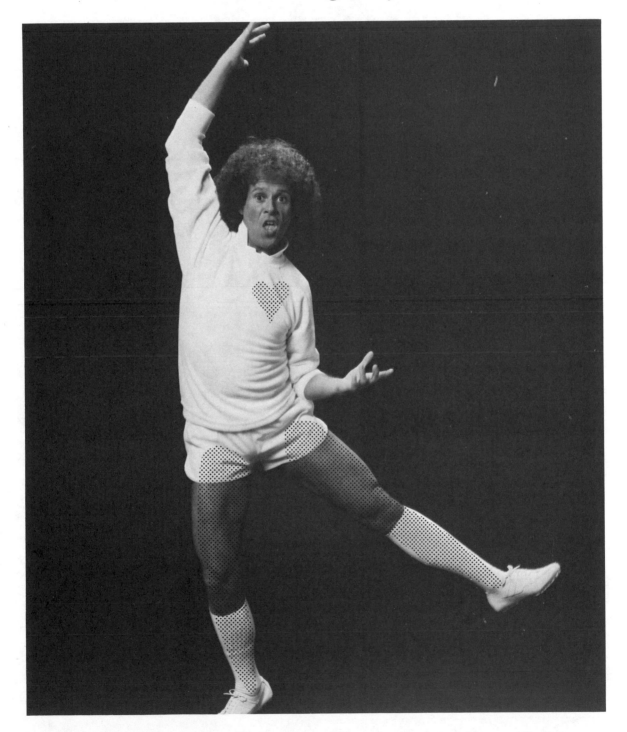

1. As your left leg kicks to the left side, your right arm goes up, with your fingers pointing up, and your left arm goes down.

2. Alternate sides.

H8 Knees Up

Position: standing, shoulders back.

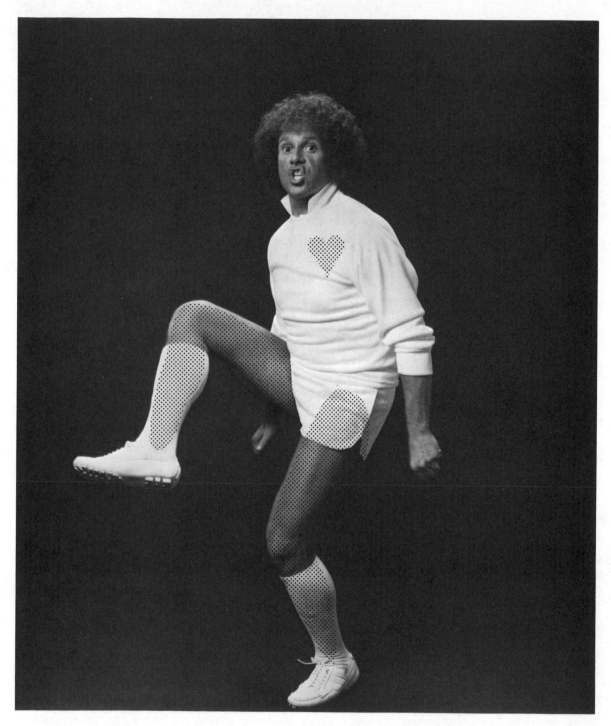

1. While running in place, bring your knees up as high as you can (one at a time, please).

H9 Heel Kicks

Position: standing, back straight, tummy in.

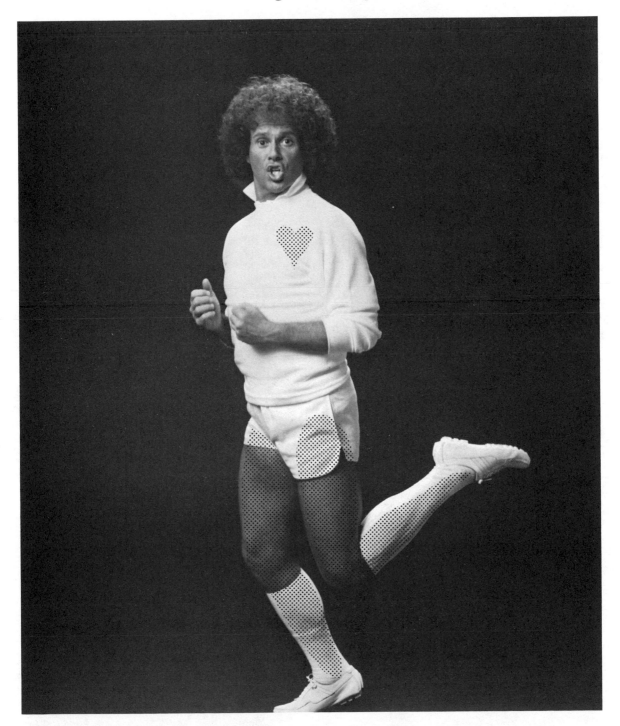

1. Kick your left heel back to touch your tushy, then kick your right heel back to touch your tushy.

2. Continue to alternate sides.

H10 Jumping Jacks

Position: standing, tummy in, legs together.

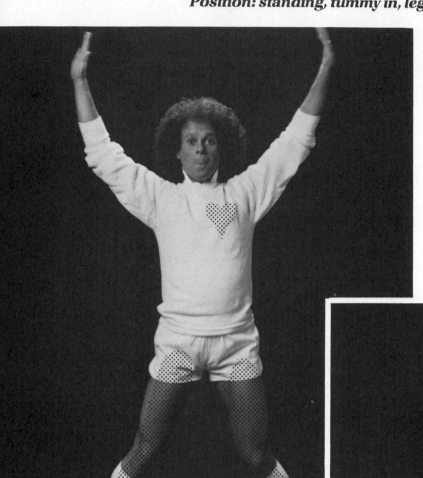

1. As you jump and open your legs bring your arms up overhead.

2. As you jump again bring your arms down and your legs together.

3. Be sure to bend your knees as you come down so there's no jolt or injury to your back and no strain on your knees.

H11 Jumping Jack Side Lunges

Position: standing, tummy in, legs apart.

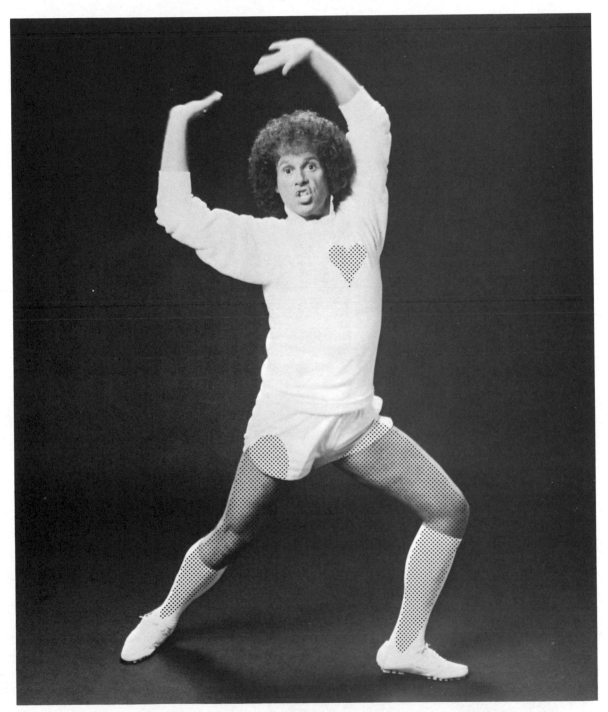

1. **As you jump bring your arms up overhead and bring your legs together.**

2. **As you jump again jump into a lunge position—one leg straight, the other leg bent.**

3. **Continue to alternate sides.**

H12 Jumping Rope

Position: standing, back straight, tummy in.

1. With your legs together, jump as if you were jumping rope.

2. Rotate your wrists as if you were rotating a jump rope.

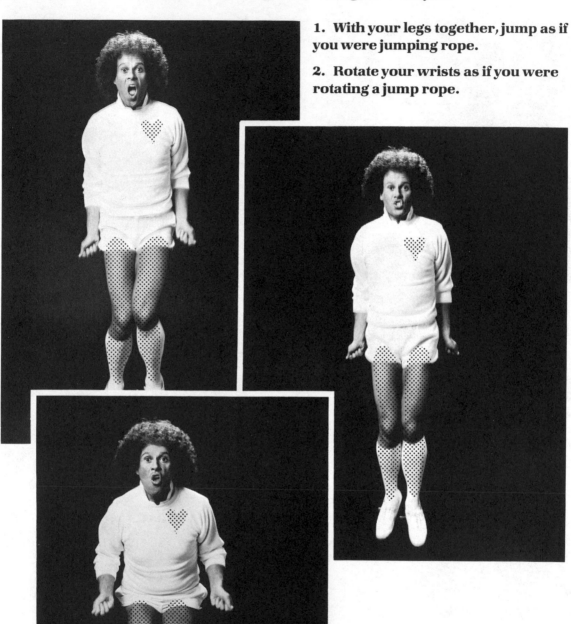

H13 Hops

Position: standing, back straight, tummy in.

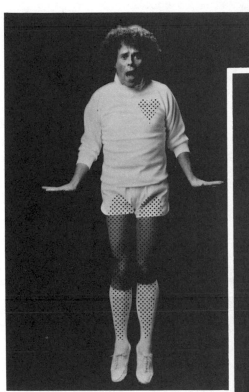

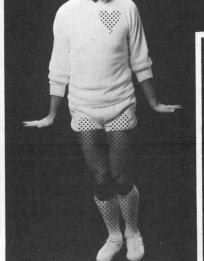

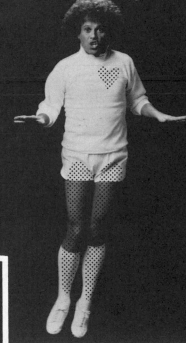

1. **Hop forward twice.**
2. **Hop back twice.**
3. **Hop right twice.**
4. **Hop left twice.**

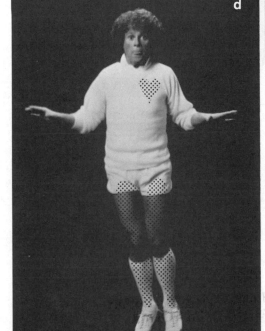

6

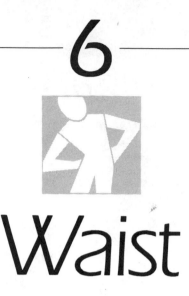

Waist

A Short History of Waists

Waists were invented by God when He created Eve. You've heard of leg men and breast men? Well, God loved waists. He also realized, after he'd made Adam, that if women were going to bear children, they would need a little more room in the equipment, so He went back to the drawing board, did some more very civil engineering, and invented waists. Waists are a direct result of the wider pelvic girdles that women must have in order to carry and deliver children. Men don't particularly have waists, because their bodies are narrower. Waists go in only because hips go out.

Sometime thereafter life got more difficult for milady. Catherine de Médicis decreed that no woman in the court could have a waist larger than sixteen inches. Of course, women were smaller then. Scarlett O'Hara railed when Mammy could tighten her corset to provide only an eighteen-inch waist. Modern woman took a look at the Miss America manual and decreed that her bust and hips should measure the same number of inches and that her waist should be ten inches smaller. (Thus 36-26-36 would be an acceptable figure.)

The liberated woman wears no corset and seldom checks her Miss America manual, so waists have become a little more relaxed. A waist that measures over twenty-four inches is not considered an embarrassment. In fact, the modern woman is more concerned that her stomach and abdomen be flat rather than that her waist fit a prescribed definition of small.

Men, on the other hand, have no waist, because their pelvic girdle is half a head smaller than a woman's. Blue jeans were devised to sit on the hips to continue the smooth line of the body. What happens? A guy gains weight and puts on love handles, so he has tires cascading over his Calvins in a manner that would make Brooke blush. How did he get so heavy? What is middle-age spread? Where did his girlish waist go?

All that fat is a result of lack of exercise. (Overeating helped, too.) Fat cells have multiplied in large glumps in bands on top of the abdominal muscles and under the skin. The skin has actually had to stretch to accommodate the fat cells, so tires build up around the middle and love handles build up in tiers.

100

W1 Side Crawls—Out

Position: standing, feet slightly apart, back straight.

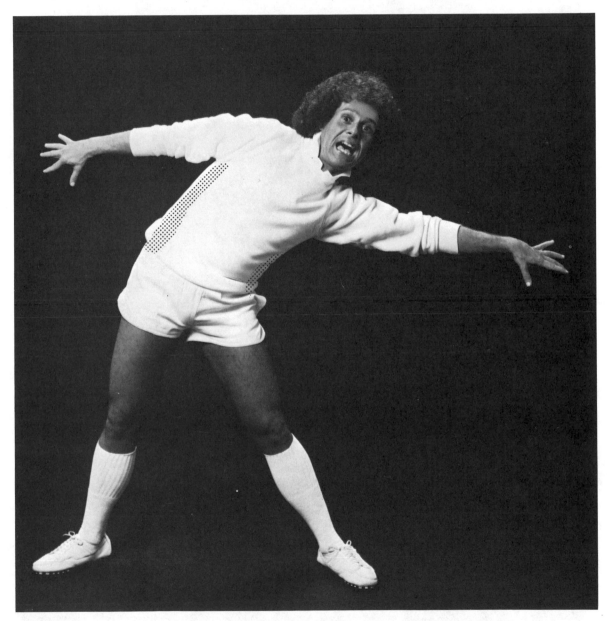

1. Lean to the left while you keep your hips tight and straight, so that you bend only at the waist.

2. Stretch your upper body to the left, extending your left arm straight out to the side while at the same time raising your right elbow up to the level of your right shoulder.

3. Alternate sides.

4. Be sure to hold in those abdominal muscles and to keep your buttocks tucked in, or you'll hurt your lower back.

W2 Side Crawls—Down

Position: standing, feet slightly apart, back straight.

1. Lean to the left while you keep your hips tight and straight, so that you bend only at the waist.

2. Stretch your upper body to the left, sliding your left arm down your body, then slide it up your body while raising your left elbow to the level of your right shoulder.

3. Alternate sides.

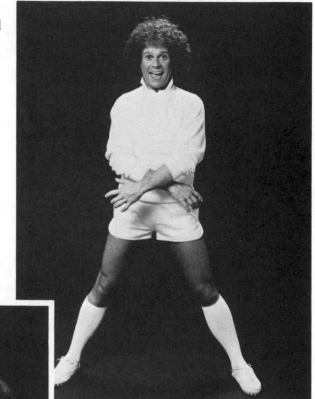

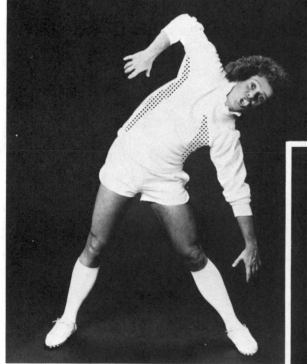

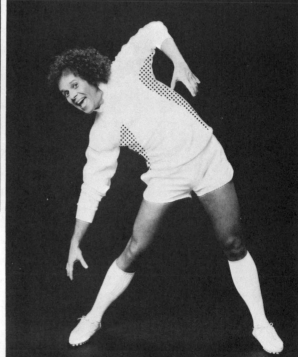

W3 Side Stretches

Position: standing, feet slightly apart, shoulders back.

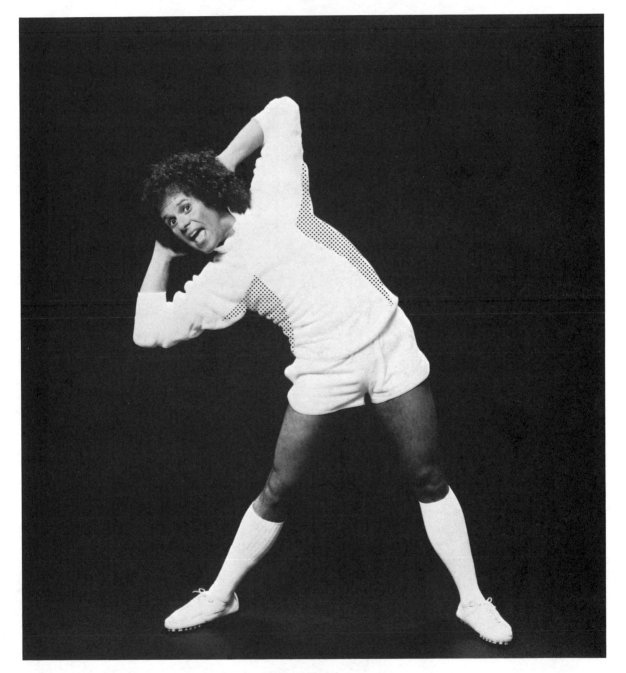

1. **Lace hands behind your head.**

2. **Bend from side to side, bending only at the waist.**

W4 Side Slide Stretches

Position: standing, feet slightly apart.

1. With back straight and shoulders back, slide your right arm down the right side of your body while you raise your left arm up.

2. Alternate sides.

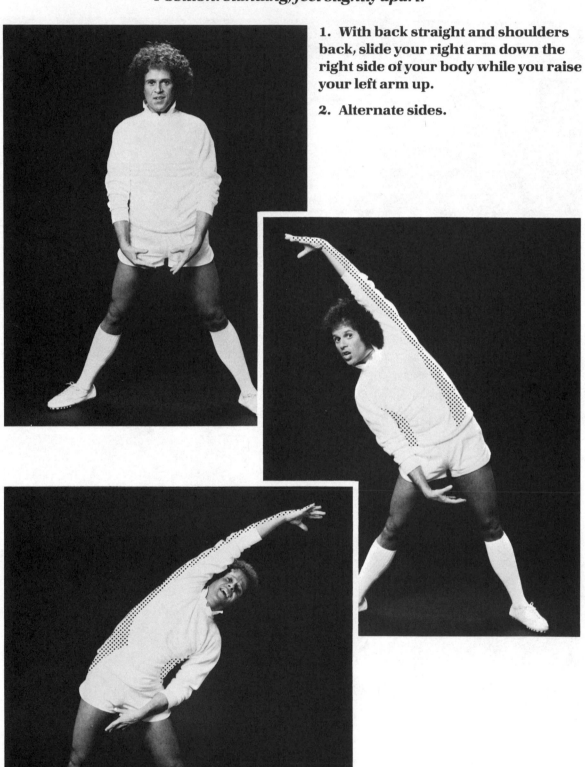

W5 Reaches

Position: standing, feet slightly apart.

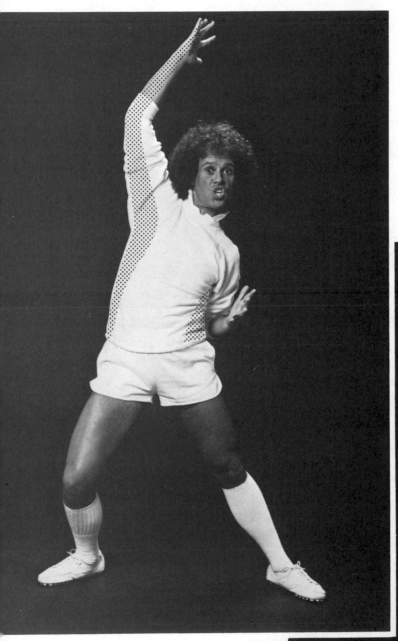

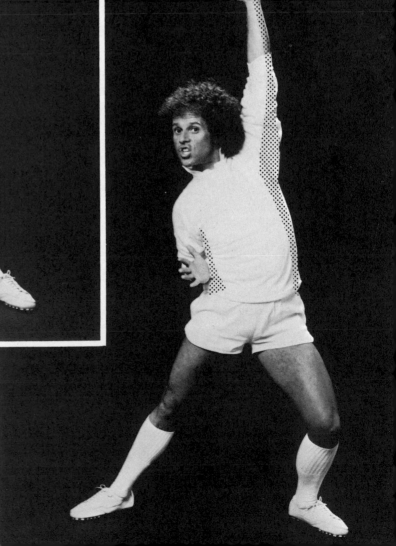

1. Bend right knee and reach up with right arm.

2. Lean into the reach, arching your arm overhead.

3. Alternate sides.

W6 Double Arm Side Stretches

Position: standing, feet slightly apart.

1. Raise both arms up overhead, keeping them close to your ears.

2. Bending from the waist, bend to the right, then to the left.

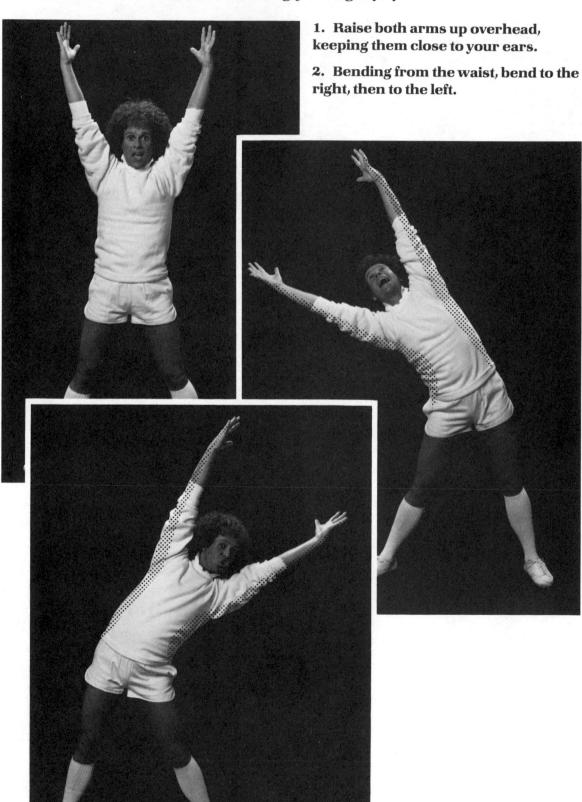

W7 Waist Twists

Position: standing, feet slightly apart, shoulders back.

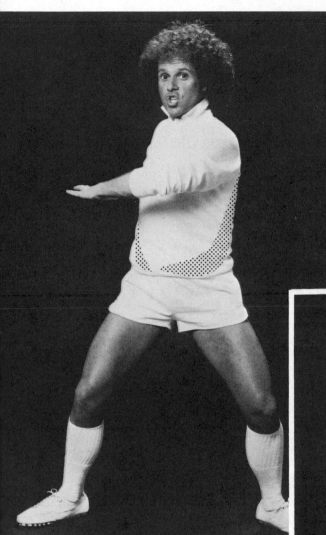

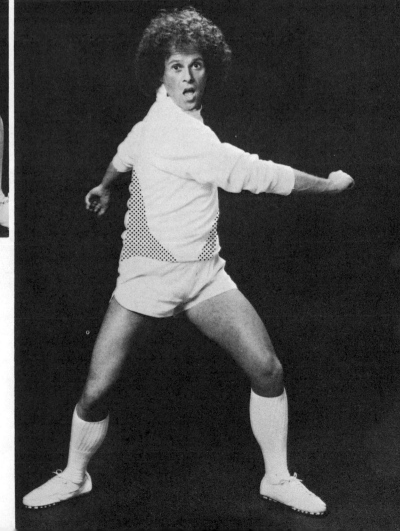

1. Bend your knees and put your arms out in front of you, with elbows bent.

2. Twist your whole upper torso to the right as far as you can.

3. Bring your body back to the front.

4. Alternate sides.

5. You should feel this in your waist.

W8 Elbow to Knee

Position: standing, feet slightly apart.

1. Touch your right elbow to your left knee while bending and twisting at your waist. The knee on the leaning side can bend while the other knee stays straight.

2. Alternate sides.

3. You should feel this in the sides of your waist.

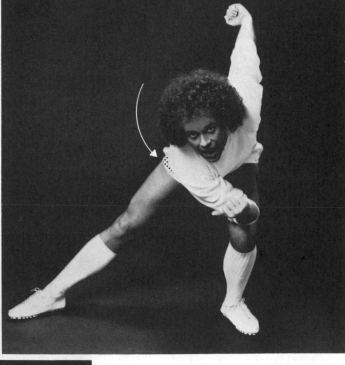

W9 Elbow to Ankle

Position: standing, feet slightly apart.

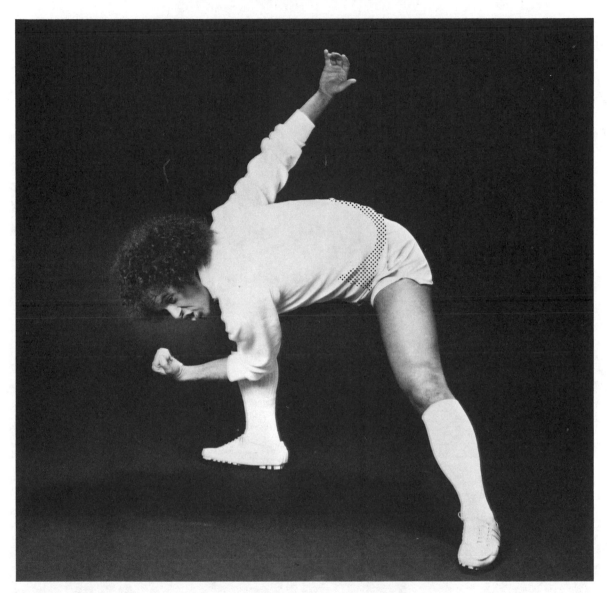

1. Touch your left elbow to your right ankle while bending and twisting at the waist.

2. Bend the knee of the leg you are touching, keeping the other one straight.

3. Alternate sides.

W10 Waist Squats

Position: standing, feet slightly apart, knees bent.

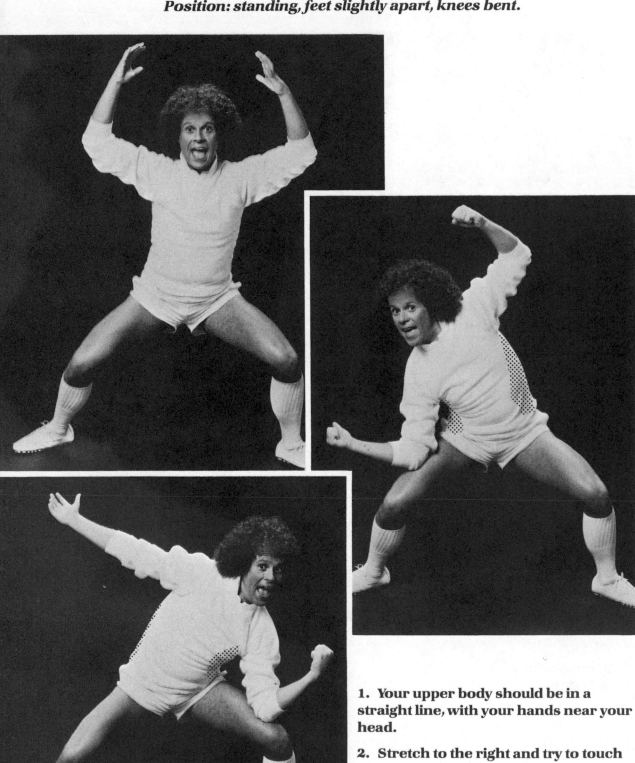

1. Your upper body should be in a
    straight line, with your hands near your
    head.

2. Stretch to the right and try to touch
    your right hip with your right elbow.

3. Alternate sides.

W11 Sliding Rib Cage

Position: standing, feet slightly apart.

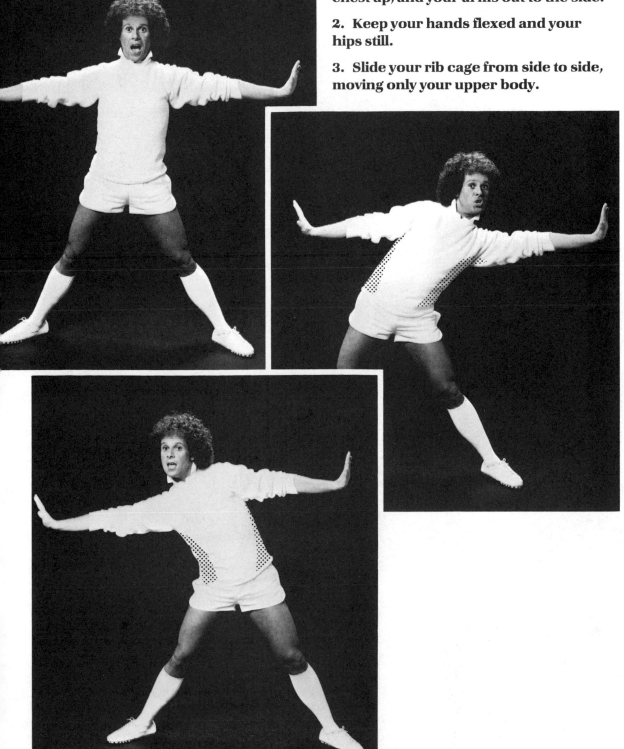

1. Keep your shoulders back, your chest up, and your arms out to the side.

2. Keep your hands flexed and your hips still.

3. Slide your rib cage from side to side, moving only your upper body.

W12 Hip Swings

Position: standing, feet slightly apart.

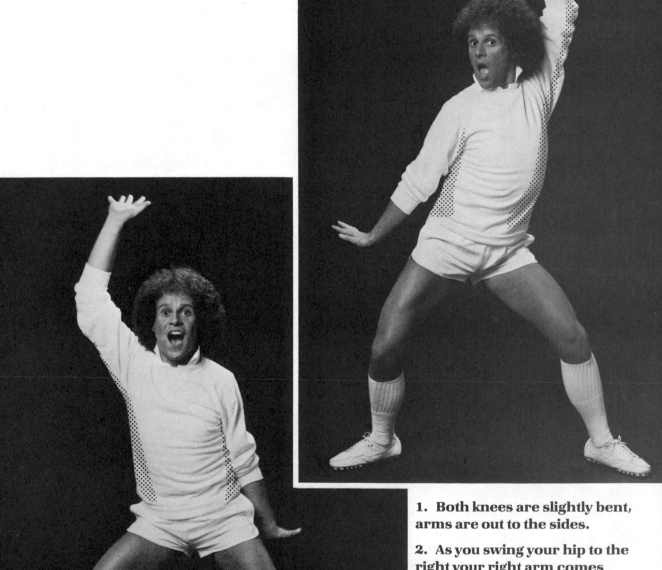

1. Both knees are slightly bent, arms are out to the sides.

2. As you swing your hip to the right your right arm comes down to meet it and your left arm swings up, then as you swing your hip to the left your left arm comes down to the left hip as the right arm swings up.

3. Alternate sides.

W13 Punches

Position: standing, feet slightly apart, knees bent.

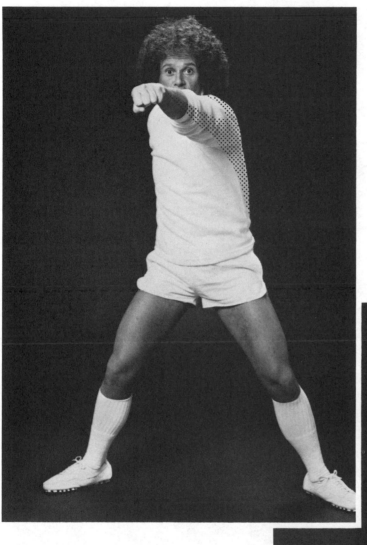

1. Lift your arms out in front of you and make fists.

2. Punch into the air while you twist at the waist, left, right, left, right, etc.

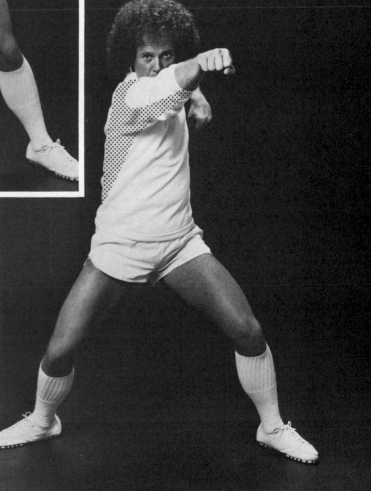

W14 Hands on Shoulders Twists

Position: standing, feet slightly apart, knees bent.

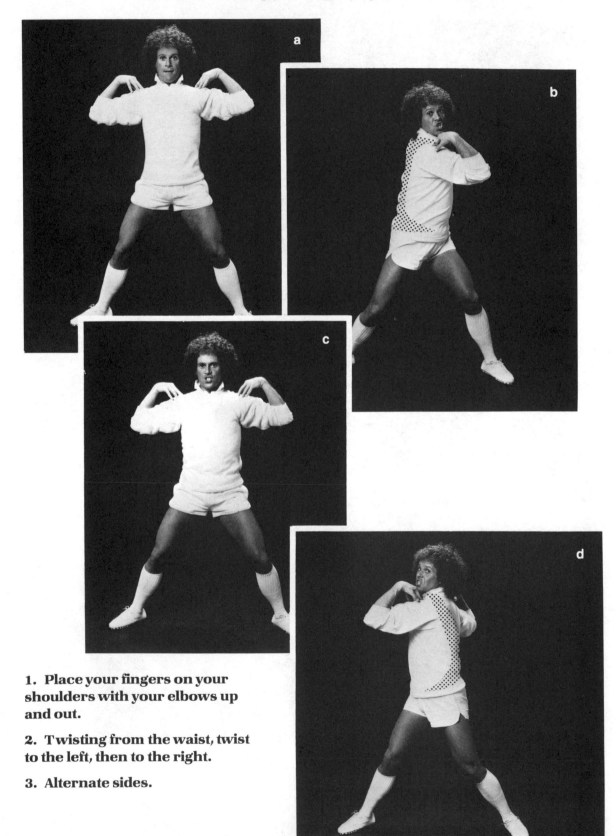

1. Place your fingers on your
shoulders with your elbows up
and out.

2. Twisting from the waist, twist
to the left, then to the right.

3. Alternate sides.

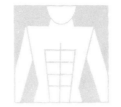

7

Stomach and Abdominals

Tummy Bummers

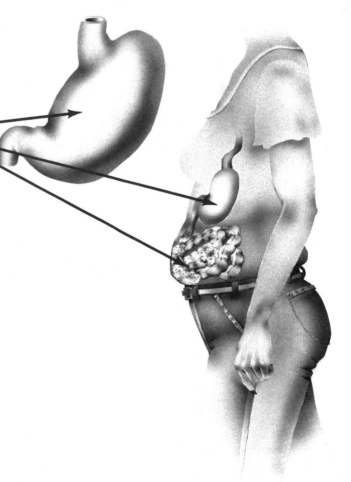

Go ahead. Do it. Put this book down and touch your stomach.

Yep, that's what I thought. You think the area between your belly button and your private parts is your stomach. Well, it's not!

So step this way for a little anatomy lesson.

This is your stomach.

It fits here in your body.

This is not your stomach.

The sag in your belly is caused by weak abdominal muscles (see page 116) or fatty buildup over your intestinal tract.

The real stomach can expand in order to make room for all the food you've been eating and can actually shrink over a period of time if not enough food comes its way. Yet, the size of the stomach has little to do with whether or not you are "fat" in that area. It's the buildup of fat cells between the intestines and your skin that makes you look fat. So, to keep your stomach and abdomen flat (the goal of every man, woman, and child over the age of twelve), you need to prevent the fat cells from moving in and making baby fat cells. By strengthening the abdominal muscles you can accomplish this goal.

The Abdominals

The muscles that make your waist waspish and your stomach flat are called the abdominals, and there are four of them:

- rectus abdominus
- external obliques
- internal obliques
- transverse abdominus.

If you're dying to look great in a bathing suit, take up belly dancing professionally, or knock out your lover when you take off your flannel granny gown, exercise in this area is a must. If you're into more fundamental activities like getting out of bed in the morning, sitting in a car, standing up straight, and preventing lower backache, the abdominals are also a team that should be exercised. And if you happen to suffer from menstrual cramps, exercise again can bail you out. (See page 266.)

Your abdominals are also vitally important in pushing out a bowel movement and giving birth to a baby, so if you're planning on having children, strong muscles before impregnation will provide a more comfortable pregnancy and an easier delivery.

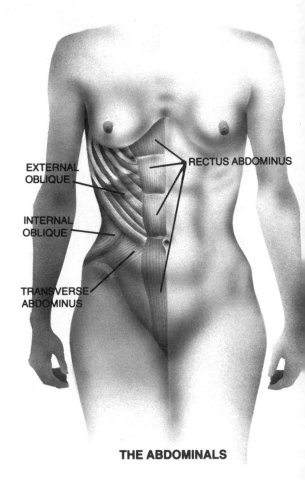

EXTERNAL OBLIQUE

RECTUS ABDOMINUS

INTERNAL OBLIQUE

TRANSVERSE ABDOMINUS

THE ABDOMINALS

Pot Bellies Are for Stoves

Pot bellies come in all shapes and sizes, but I like to see them only when they are attached to Franklin stoves and are made out of cast iron. You see pot bellies, unfortunately, on men and women and even on children. Sometimes the person is overweight and the pot belly is only one of many problems. Often the person has a relatively good figure, except for that little pot.

People who have pot bellies have generally let their exercise programs go to pot, so their sagging muscles create what looks like a little pot or pouch. Pot bellies usually begin, like volcanoes, under the surface, years before they actually show. The most common example is the woman who was always slim to begin with, so she did no exercising after her three children were born. (Okay, so you hate her. Wait—she'll get hers.) After the third child and her thirty-fifth birthday, she "suddenly" developed a pot belly. Had she tightened up after the birth of her first child and continued exercising steadily thereafter, she never would have developed the "sudden" pot belly. Now she'll have a lot of trouble getting rid of it. (No fair going to Brazil for a tummy tuck.)

Pot bellies work like this:

1. You lack exercise, so your abdominals are weak.

2. You eat until you feel full, which gives you lots of room, because your abdominals are too weak to give you a warming tinge. (Sounds like catch-22 already, doesn't it?)

3. You eat until you are uncomfortable, which is a lot of food and more than what you actually need.

4. Your stomach begins to bulge, and you think you should cut back on what you eat, but it's hard to leave the table hungry. You never realize that exercise will tighten those muscles and make you feel full sooner, thus eliminating the round-and-round tin circles aspect of this problem.

My Tummy

An Essay by Milton Simmons

My Tummy is my friend. I can rest my arms on it. I can bounce pencils off it. I can play Rocket Ship to Mars with my belly button as a launchpad. I love my waist. Whenever I go on a weight loss plan, I measure my waist first. Tops and bottoms aren't as important as waists. Belts are nice, unless your waist is seventy-five inches big. Then you can't find a belt to fit you. I wonder who invented belts. Probably Benjamin Franklin or Thomas A. Edison. They invented everything else. God did not invent belts, or Eve would have been wearing one—probably made out of snakeskin. Even though my waist is my friend, I am trying to shrink it. Yesterday I bought Waste Away, a new product that makes you skinny. It's a combination of Elmer's Glue-All and Ben-Gay. Boy, does it tickle. It has a sponge applicator, and I painted the goop on my body. That's why I am writing this essay from the hospital.

Keeping the Stomach Flat

Save your money. You don't have to rush out and buy one of those fast-read quick tummy-toner books. Once you're in shape, all you need to do is tuck those footsies under the bed frame and put in a hundred sit-ups a morning (before breakfast).

If you haven't been exercising those abdominal muscles for about twenty years, let me see, you owe about 36,500 sit-ups a year, times twenty years. . . . You owe your body 730,000 sit-ups. Do you want that on your tombstone?

Without a doubt the hardest part of this book will be doing these stomach exercises and sit-ups. But I guarantee, if you are faithful for thirty days, you'll see a difference. And it'll be easier after that. Easy skiing, I promise.

People Always Hold Their Stomachs In When:

- trying on clothes.
- they walk by a mirror.
- they meet someone for the first time.
- their husband's ex-wife walks by.
- the principal of the school asks them to stop by the office.
- the Academy Award for Best Actor is announced.
- they remember their wedding day.

You cannot hold your stomach in for the rest of your life. Work it off, or live with it.

S1 Tummy Warmers

Position: on mat, sitting up.

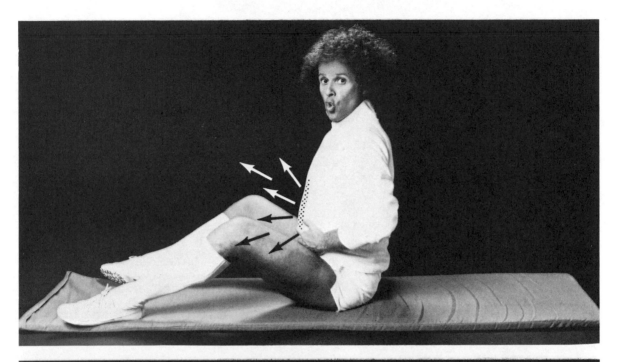

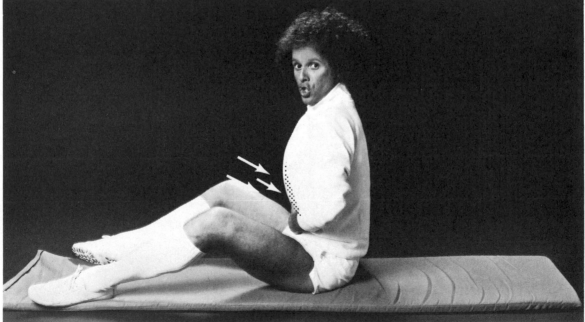

1. While sitting comfortably, practice breathing for sit-ups.

2. Place your hands on your abdomen. Inhale—expand your abdomen out. Exhale—pull your abdomen in.

3. Your knees should be bent with your feet apart on the floor.

S2 *Upper Abdominal Lifts*

Position: on mat, lying down, knees bent.

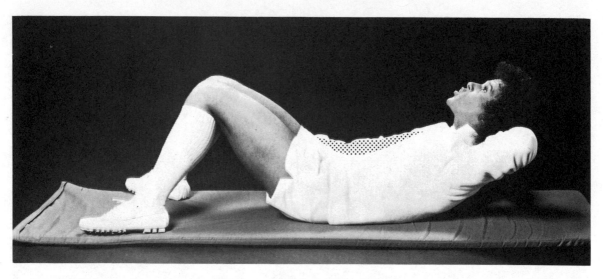

1. Feet are apart, knees are together, hands are held behind your head.

2. Keeping your elbows locked into position, lift yourself up from the waist, bringing your shoulders off the mat.

3. Lower yourself back down.

S3 Single Leg Lifts

Position: on mat, lying down, knees bent.

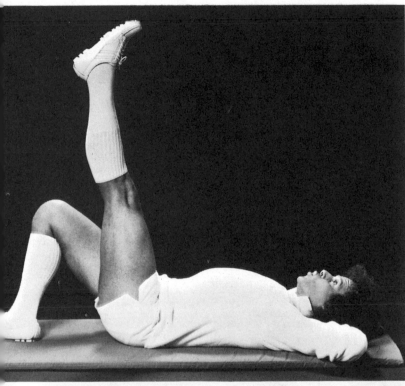

1. Lift your left leg up toward the ceiling with your foot flexed.

2. With your elbows out to the sides, bring your chin toward the leg you are lifting without moving that leg.

3. Alternate sides.

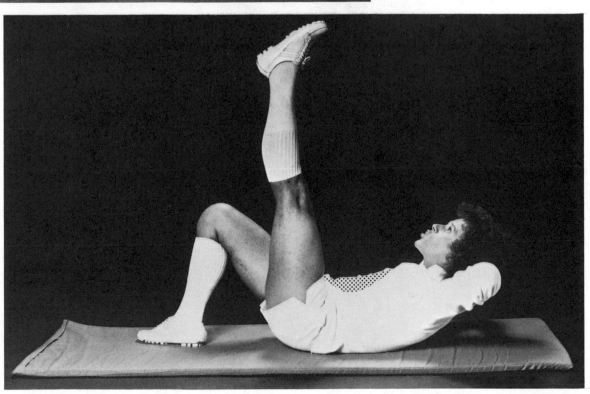

S4 Double Leg Lifts

Position: on mat, lying down.

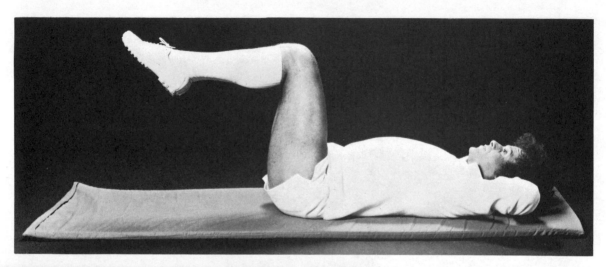

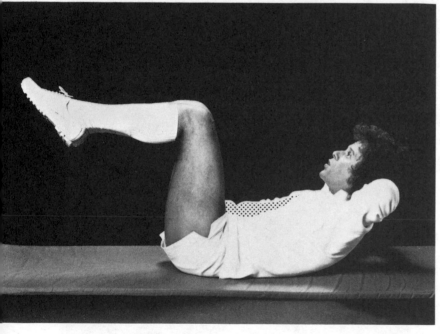

1. Bring your knees up with your feet flexed. (Imagine your legs are resting on a chair seat.) Hands are held behind your head.

2. Bring your chin toward your legs, then lower yourself back down.

3. Be sure not to arch your back.

S5 Crunch Twists

Position: on mat, lying down.

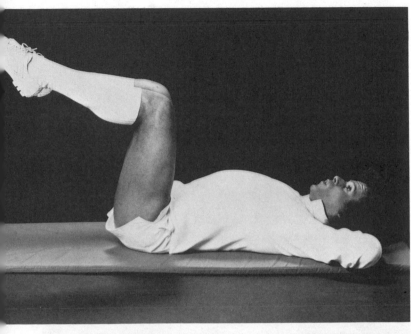

1. Bring your knees up with your feet flexed. (Imagine your legs are resting on a chair seat.) Hands are held behind your head.

2. As you sit up twist to the left from the shoulders, touch your right elbow to your left knee, lower yourself down, then as you sit up again twist to the right, touching your left elbow to your right knee.

3. If you are very advanced, do this with your shoulders off the ground.

4. Alternate sides.

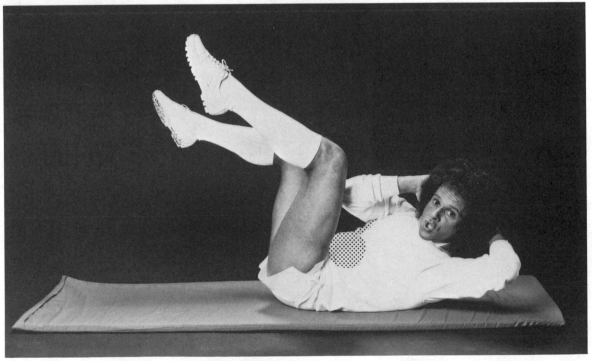

S6 Crunch Twists—Straight Legs

Position: on mat, lying down.

1. Bring your legs straight into the air with your feet flexed. Hands are held behind your head.

2. As you sit up twist to the left from the shoulders, touch your right elbow to your left knee, lower yourself down, then as you sit up again twist to the right, touching your left elbow to your right knee.

3. Alternate sides.

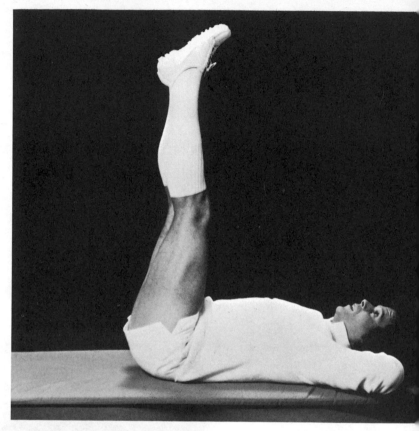

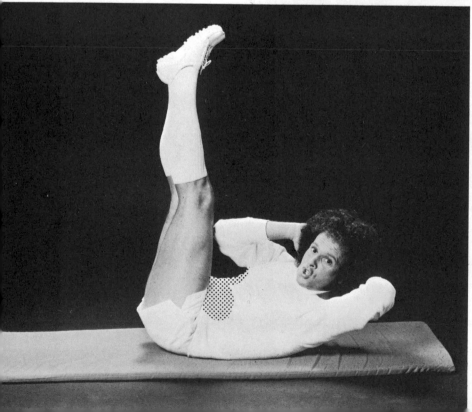

S7 Lower Abdominal Reaches

Position: on mat, lying down, legs apart.

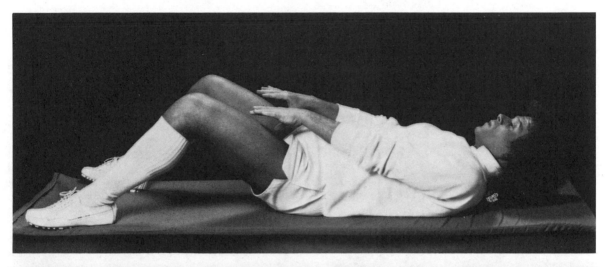

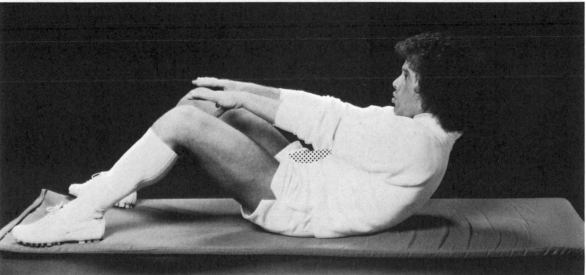

1. With your feet on the floor and your knees bent, sit up and reach through your legs, bouncing back and forth.

S8 Lower Abdominal Reaches— Feet Up

Position: on mat, lying down, legs apart.

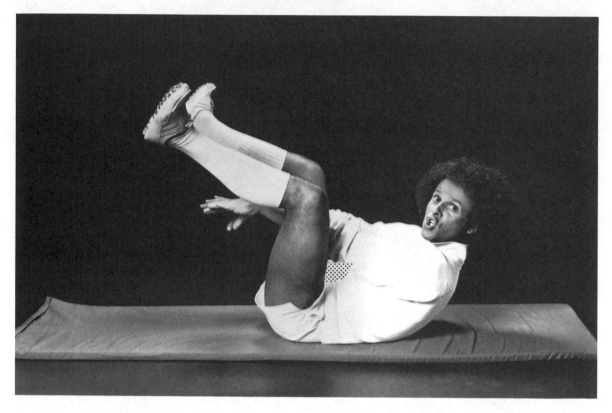

1. With your feet up in the air and your knees bent (as if your legs were resting on a chair seat), sit up and reach through your legs, bouncing back and forth.

S9 One Leg Reaches—Up

Position: on mat, lying down.

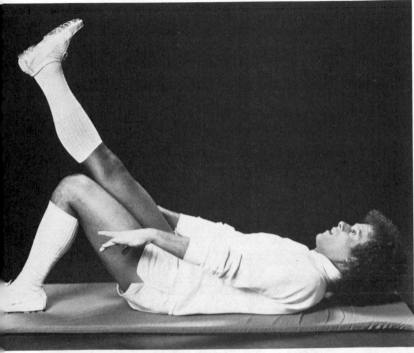

1. With one leg bent at the knee and foot on the floor, bring the other leg straight up in the air.

2. Arms are alongside the body.

3. Tuck your chin in toward your chest and reach out, lifting your shoulders.

4. Alternate legs.

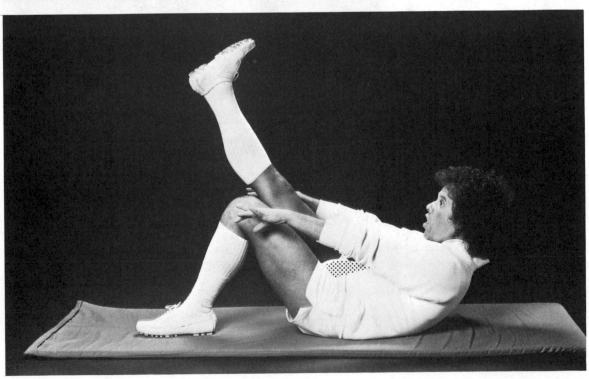

S10 One Leg Reaches—Out

Position: on mat, lying down.

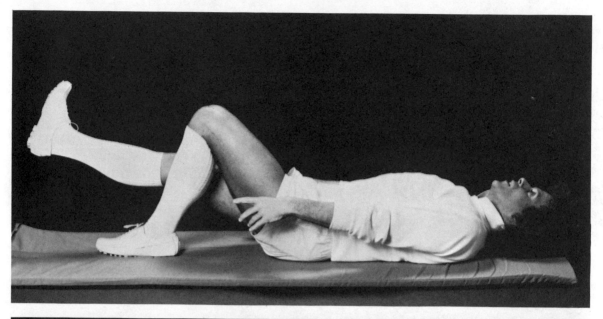

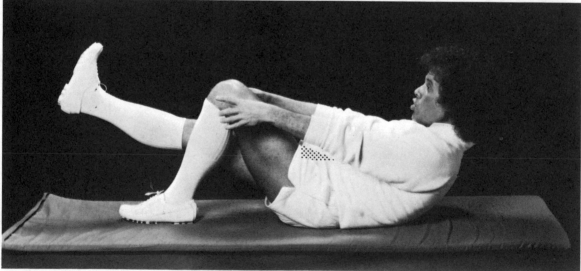

1. One leg is bent at the knee with the foot on the floor. The other leg is straight out parallel to the mat with the foot flexed a few inches off the floor.

2. Arms are alongside the body.

3. Reach down the length of your body as you sit up, making sure your lower back is on the ground.

S11 Crunch Reaches

Position: on mat, lying down, knees bent.

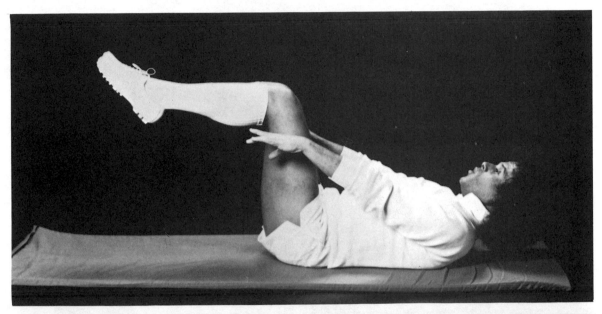

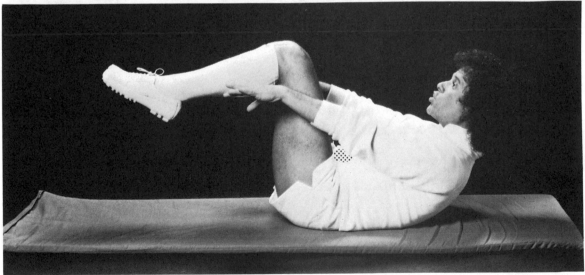

1. Knees are together, feet are together. Lift them about two feet off the ground into the chair position.

2. Arms are alongside the body and will reach out along the body as you sit up.

3. Sit up, lie down, sit up, etc.

S12 Straight Leg Crunch Reaches

Position: on mat, lying down.

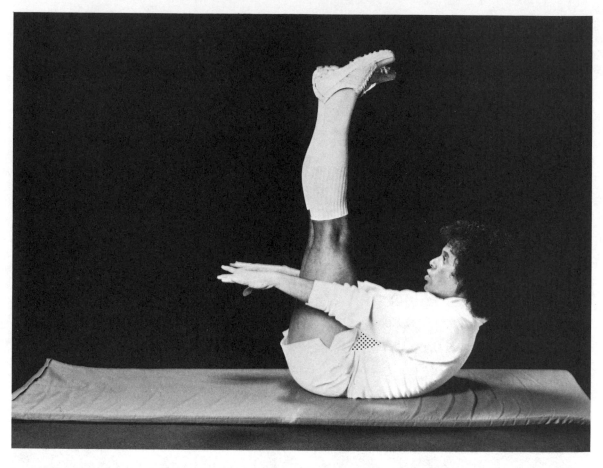

1. **Lift both legs straight up in the air, keeping your arms alongside your body.**

2. **Reach arms straight alongside your body as you sit up.**

S13 Hands Under Bent Leg Extensions

Position: on mat, lying down.

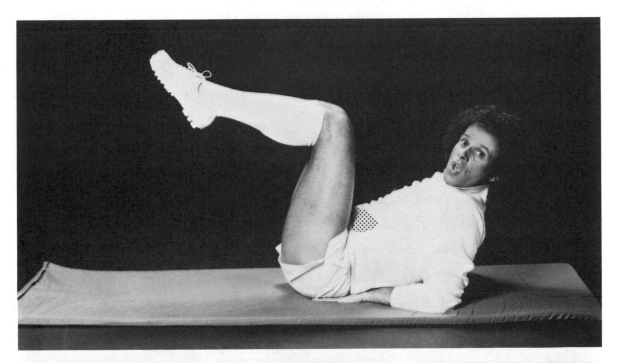

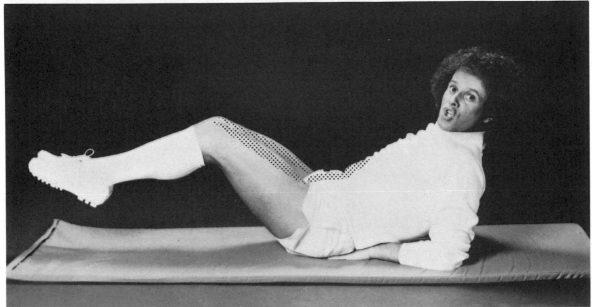

1. With arms up on your elbows, place hands under your tush.

2. Bend your legs in the imaginary chair position.

3. Extend legs with toes pointed toward the floor, but don't touch the ground.

4. Bring your legs back toward your chin.

S14 Straight Leg Extensions

Position: on mat, lying down.

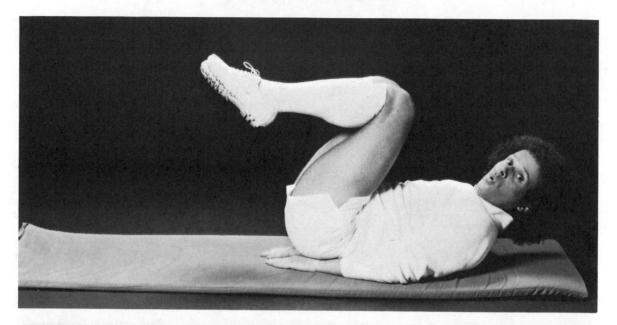

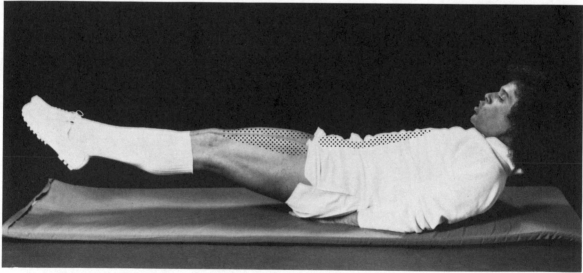

1. **Place hands under tush. Bend legs in imaginary chair position.**

2. **Extend legs with toes pointed toward the floor, straightening them all the way.**

3. **Bring your legs back toward your face.**

S15 Scissors

Position: on mat, lying down.

1. Place hands under tush and raise both legs straight up in the air.

2. Bring right leg up and left one down, like a pair of scissors.

3. Alternate legs.

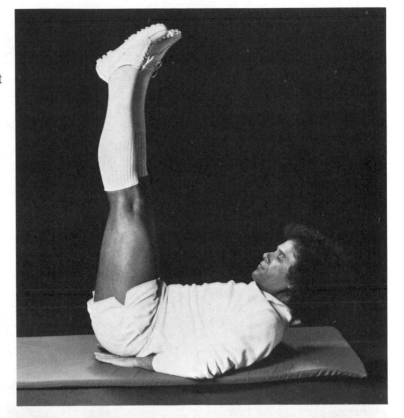

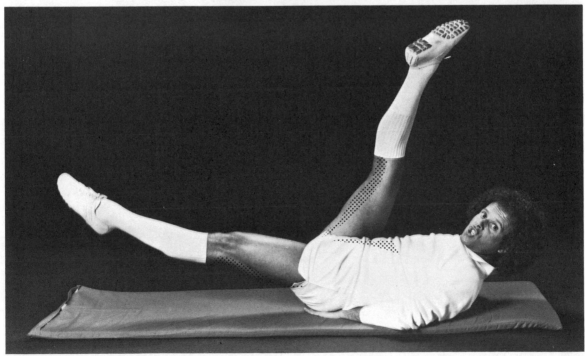

S16 One Leg Up—One Leg Out—Hold

Position: on mat, lying down.

1. Place arms at your sides.

2. Bring right leg straight up, flex foot, and bring left leg out to the left side and point toe. Hold.

3. Keep lower back on the ground and shoulders and head up.

4. If you are a beginner, you can do this by having one leg bent at the knee on the mat, then bringing the other leg into the air and holding it.

5. You will feel this in your stomach and the backs of your legs.

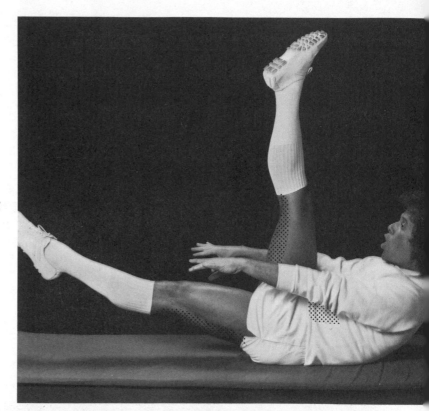

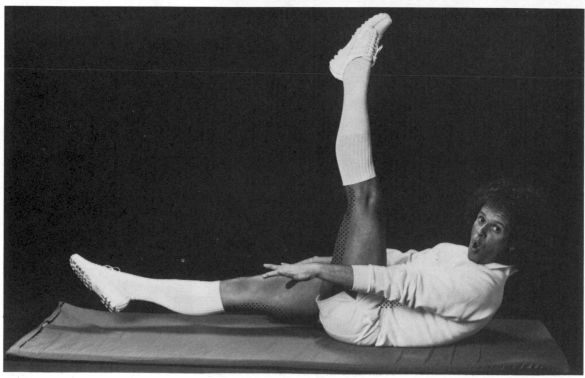

S17 Back Breaks

Position: on mat, lying down.

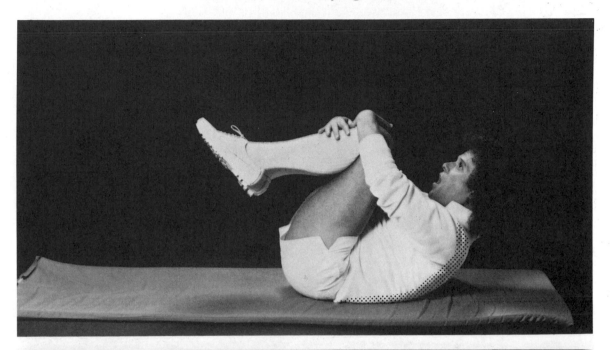

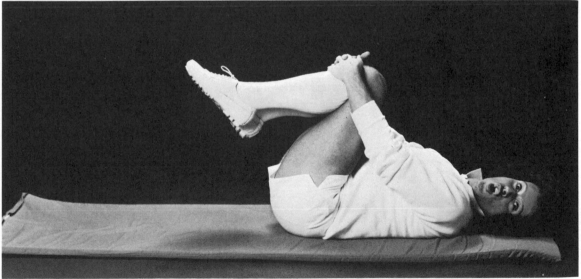

1. Lying on your back with your head and shoulders up, grab your knees to your chest. Release, extend, with head and shoulders on floor, and return to chest.

S18 Knee Grabs

Position: on mat, lying down.

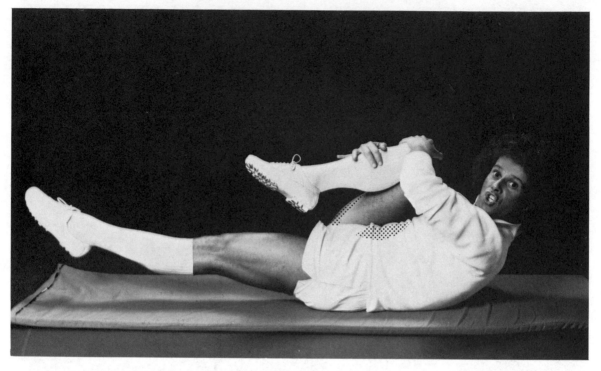

1. Keeping your head and shoulders up, grab one knee to your chest with elbows out to the sides.

2. Alternate knees, pointing your feet. Neither foot should touch the ground.

S19 Bicycles

Position: on mat, lying down.

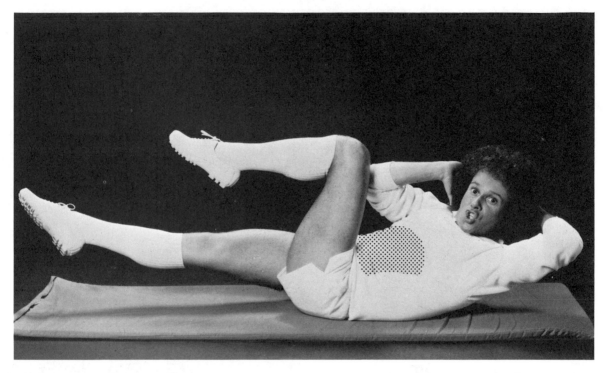

1. **Place hands behind your head.**

2. **Bring opposite elbow to opposite knee.**

3. **Keep lower back on the ground.**

4. **Alternate sides.**

S20 Lower Back Drops

Position: on mat, sitting up halfway.

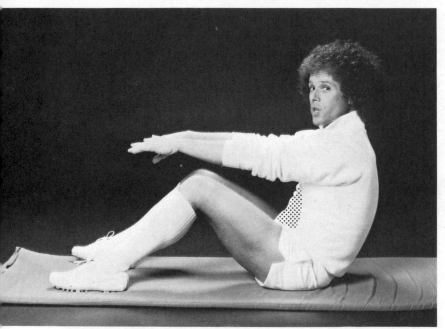

1. Legs are bent at the knee with feet flat on the ground. Back should be rounded to prevent strain.

2. Arms are straight out in front of you.

3. Pull in tummy toward back and lower your back toward the ground. Lower back should touch the ground, but your shoulders shouldn't.

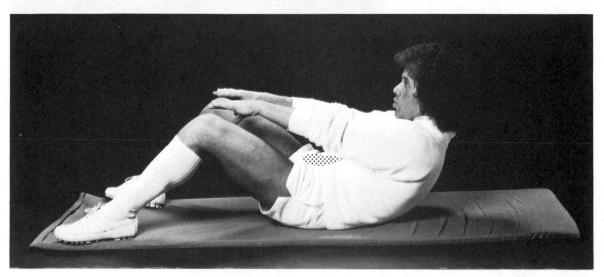

S21 Climbing Rope

Position: on mat, sitting up halfway.

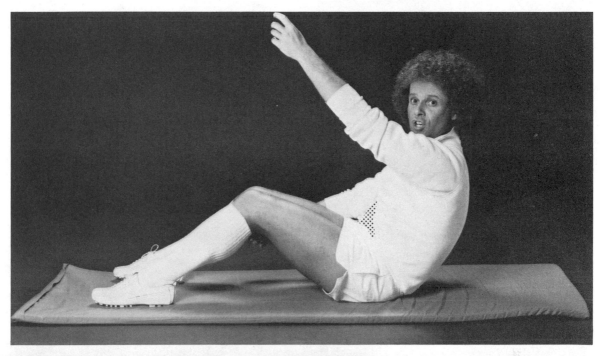

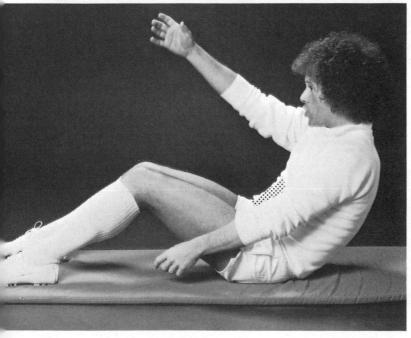

1. Feet are on the ground with knees bent and back rounded.

2. Lean halfway back and bring one arm up overhead, then the other.

3. Alternate strokes as you imitate climbing a rope. Pretend the pirates are after you and you're climbing the rigging. This is a lot like doing The Monkey while seated.

S22 Half Position Twists

Position: on mat, sitting up halfway.

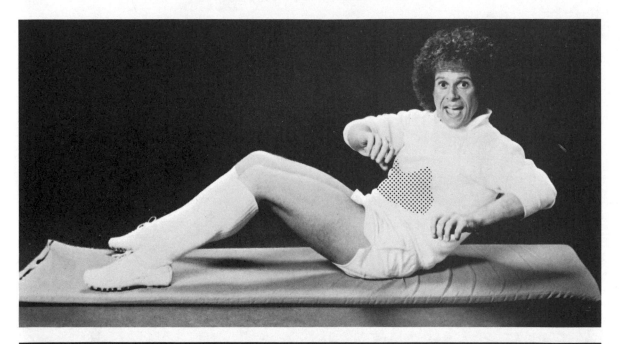

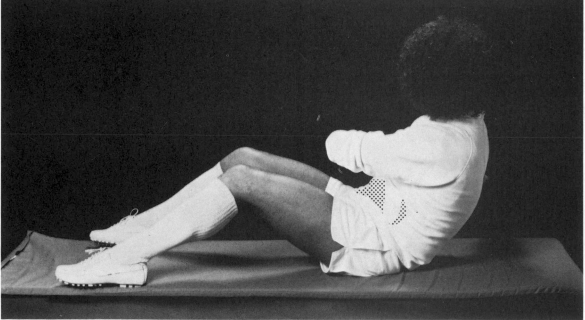

1. **Feet are on the ground with knees bent and back rounded.**

2. **Lean halfway back and twist from side to side.**

S23 *Advanced Twists*

Position: on mat, lying down.

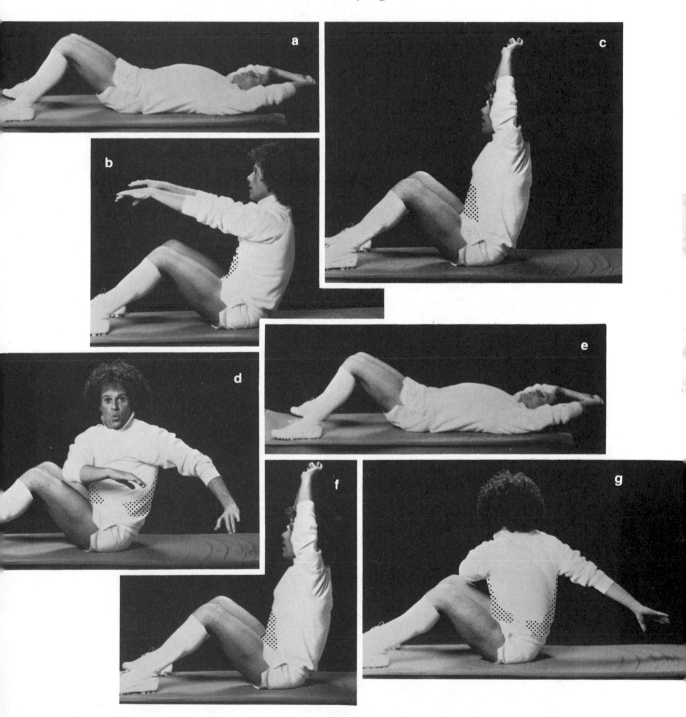

1. Feet are on the ground with knees bent and back rounded.

2. Sit up with arms straight out in front, back rounded.

3. Raise arms overhead.

4. Twist to the left, untwist, lie down, sit up, twist to the right, untwist, lie down, etc.

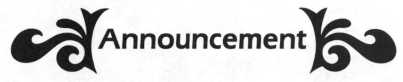# Announcement

Many people do not exercise their stomach and abdominal muscles because they think it will hurt their lower backs. This is a myth. These same exercises will also help strengthen your back.

8

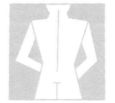

Upper and Lower Back (Posture, Too)

—Oh, My Aching Back—

Eight out of every ten people in the world (I say, that's a lot of people) will suffer from backaches at one time or another. Ninety percent of these people say they can't exercise because they have back problems. Yet, many of these aches and pains can be prevented, and most of these people should be exercising.

According to doctors, about eighty percent of all backache complaints are related to muscle strain. In other words, they could be prevented!

You can prevent back pain by doing specific exercises to strengthen back muscles and by doing these same exercises as a preliminary warmup before sports. Most sports injuries are a result of not warming up or down

properly or not being in good enough shape to actually play the sport well.

Needless to say, if you are walking around carrying extra weight, you are also putting an unnecessary burden on your back and thus causing an ache where you may be able to eliminate one. Backaches are frequent visitors to pregnant women and overweighters of any sex, because every additional pound is a load.

Posture also has a lot to do with backache. Weak muscles lead to poor posture, which leads to backache, and back again into that same old vicious cycle. Good posture is not so much a matter of pulling your shoulder blades back, but of lifting up at the lower back and holding your torso erect.

The Back

The back has come to mean the back part of the body, anywhere from the neck to the tush, but it is more appropriately divided into two parts: the upper and lower back.

From the atlas to the coccyx, there are twenty-four little vertebrae who are hoping you never injure them. It is the main function of the spinal column to support the weight of the body, head to toe. Between each vertebra is a cushion called an intervertebral disk. Thus the expression "to slip a disk" means that one of those little suckers has gone astray and is causing you severe pain. The disks serve as shock absorbers and allow the vertebrae to move in relation to each other, so you can flex and extend your spine. The disks have a high water content, and so they can be ruptured and, over the years, they can become less elastic, making it harder to move without pain.

The muscles of the back are divided into three groups: a superficial group, an intermediate group, and a deep group. (And you thought all this medical stuff was too complicated for you!)

These three groups work together to fill in the space between the spinal column and the ribs, to hold the organs beneath them in place and the body upright. The spine has about a thousand ligaments that attach the whole rigamarole to the spinal column. There are also muscles, tendons, and about one hundred fifty little joints that give you the flexibility you have. If your spinal column is in line, you'll have good posture and little back trouble. If anything goes haywire, pain sets in!

One of the best ways to protect your back is to realize what a vulnerable area it is and to protect it by strengthening it with exercise and by being good to it, as follows:

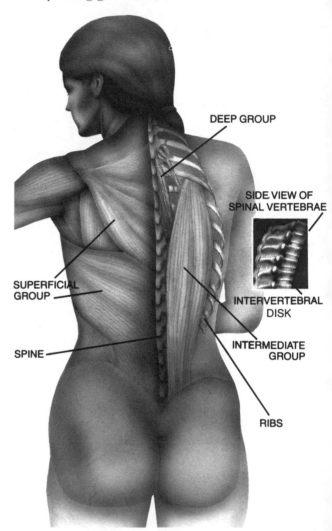

DEEP GROUP

SIDE VIEW OF SPINAL VERTEBRAE

SUPERFICIAL GROUP

INTERVERTEBRAL DISK

SPINE

INTERMEDIATE GROUP

RIBS

THE BACK MUSCLES

- DO bend at the knees, not at the waist.
- DO avoid picking up heavy loads.
- DO hold heavy objects close to your body.
- DO sleep properly. (DON'T sleep on your back with your legs straight out.)
- DO take pressure off your back by changing foot position if you are on your feet for a while.
- DO release stress so it doesn't cause back pain.
- DO sit properly, with the lower back supported.

Posture

You can have the slimmest, cutest body in the whole world, but it's going to look awful—yes, awful—if you don't have good posture to go with it. Posture is a function of the lower back, the shoulders, and the neck, but it is also a psychological matter. Look around you. People who are bent over and exhibit sagging body language have low self-esteem, are unhappy, unproud, and unconfident. People with good posture always look like they can conquer the world. Looks might not be everything, but they sure count for a lot.

I'm not going to tell you to walk around the house, balancing this book on your head to see how straight you can carry your body, but I do want you to step over to the mirror and take a look at yourself. Good posture helps the body function better, makes you look taller and slimmer, and enhances your confidence. How do you look? Are your shoulders hunched forward, rounded? Is there tension in your neck or your shoulders? Do you feel tight, mad, angry? Are your shoulder blades back or forward? Do you have a swayed back? Is your chin buried in this book or up and out?

The secret to good posture is to pretend you are of royal birth.

- Lift your head upward, to keep the crown balanced. Your eyes should be looking straight out at the crowd, your cheering people. The chin can even be slightly tilted up in a jaunty air. Don't go too high up—aim for a right angle with your throat.
- Hold your neck up and pretend that you are stretching it. This happens by itself if your crown is on and your shoulders are down.
- Pull your shoulders down away from your ears and back so they are lined up with your hip bones.
- Lift your chest up off your waist and pull in your tummy while you tuck under your buns. No one likes a royal with a big bum.
- As you are raising up your chest note that your spine lengthens and straightens by itself. Now that ermine cloak will look great on you.
- Make sure that your pelvis is tucked in and under.

Got it? Good. When a throne becomes available, I'll let you know.

The Incredible Shrinking Woman

As people get older they tend to shrink. This is not a joke. I used to think it was my imagination and I'd say to myself, "Aw, c'mon, Dickie, no one can really shrink." But now I've learned that older people really do shrink, and get this part: Women shrink faster than men.

Osteoporosis is the name of the condition in which the bones grow closer together and often become more brittle. That's why silver citizens have a greater tendency to break a wrist or a hip, why it takes so long for their breaks to heal, and why they are often bent over like commas. Even if there is no bending, there is still a settling in and a small amount of shrinking.

Osteoporosis cannot be cured once you have it. A trip to the rack will not stretch you back to your original height. (And forget about getting taller, I've been trying that for years.) BUT osteoporosis can be prevented or controlled with proper nutrition, a lot of exercises, and sometimes medical treatment by a doctor. Women are more prone to this problem after the Big Change, so doctors now think that hormone treatments may help prevent osteoporosis.

So if you're feeling lazy today, or you like that age-old excuse for not exercising—you know the one: "I've got lower backache, I can't exercise"—take a look around you and rest your eyeballs on the elderly. The ones who are the most stooped over, the ones with the worst back pains, are the ones who thought like you do. Exercise today will help prevent this terrible problem thirty or forty years from now. Don't be sorry later. Be smart now.

B1 Spinal Twists—Straddle Position

Position: sitting, legs apart.

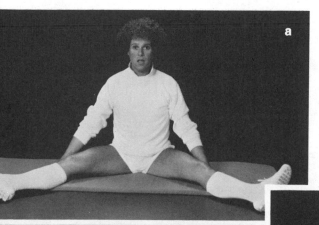

1. With your back straight, place right hand outside of left knee and raise left arm up and over your head, arching toward the right side. Reach and twist.

2. Bring both arms overhead like a butterfly, then alternate sides.

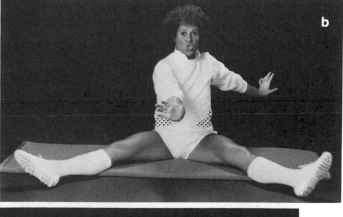

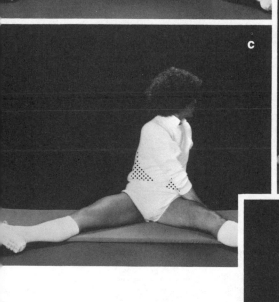

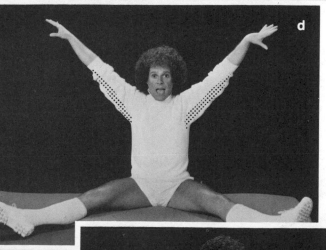

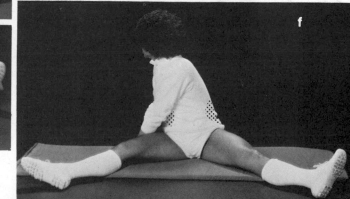

B2 Spinal Twists—Lying Down

Position: on mat, lying down.

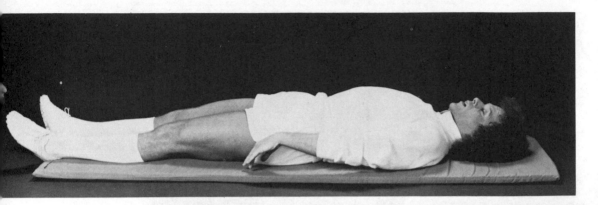

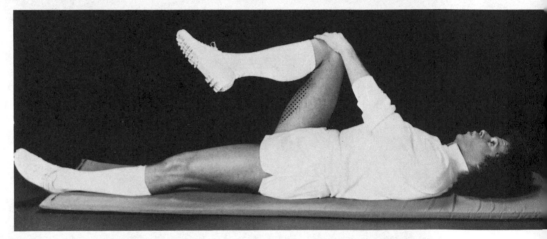

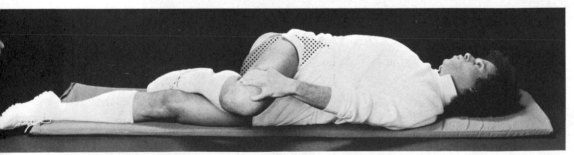

1. Arms are at your sides.

2. Leaving your left leg straight out on the mat, bend your right knee and bring your right leg across your left leg.

3. Shoulders should stay on the ground.

4. Alternate sides.

B3 Spinal Twists—Straight Leg

Position: on mat, lying down.

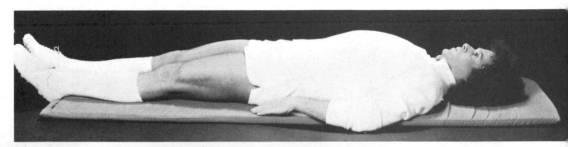

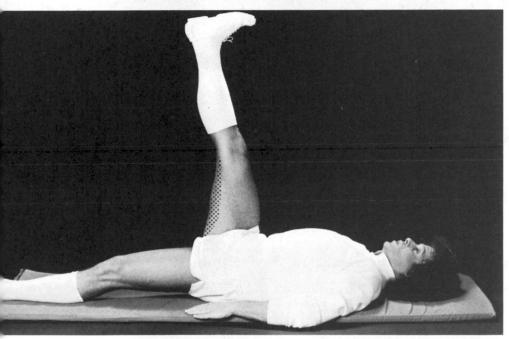

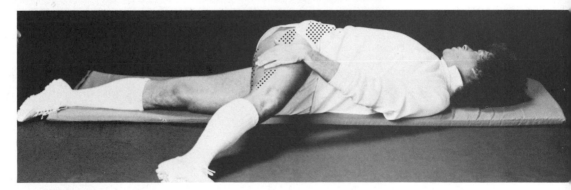

1. **Arms are at your sides.**

2. **Raise right leg straight in the air and bring it across your left leg.**

3. **Shoulders should stay on the ground.**

4. **Alternate sides.**

B4 Pelvic Push Downs

Position: on mat, lying down.

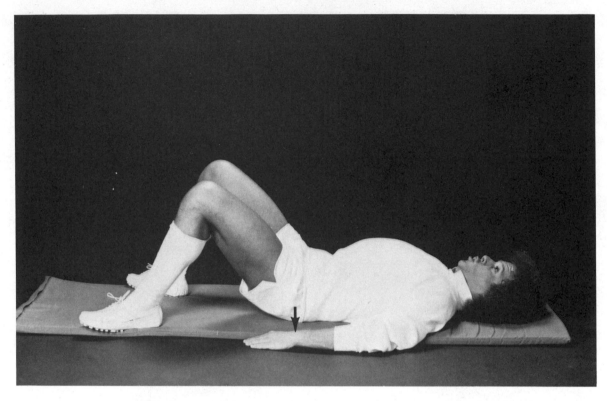

1. With knees bent, slightly raise up pelvis. Keep shoulders on the ground.

2. Push down on the pelvis while keeping buns off the ground.

B5 Froggy on the Pond

Position: on mat, lying down.

1. With shoulders and head up, put your feet together and grab them with your hands.

2. Keep knees bent and apart and use your hands to press your ankles closer to your body while lowering your back.

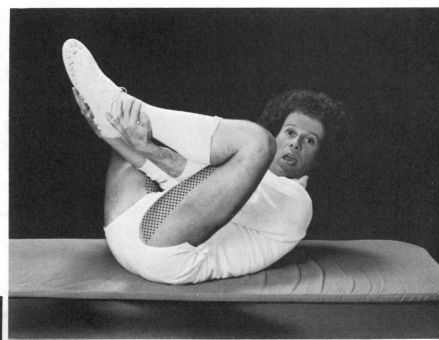

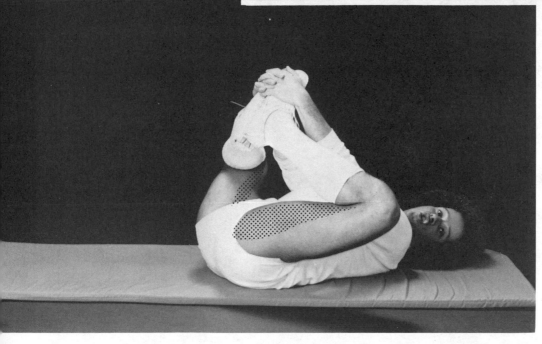

B6 Cobra

Position: on mat, lying on stomach.

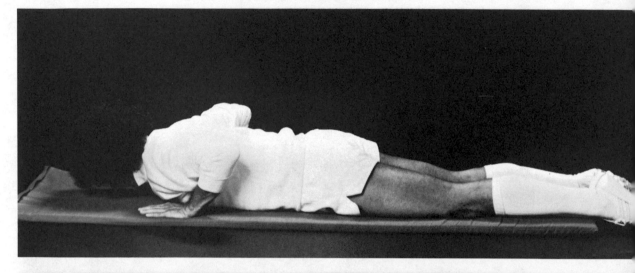

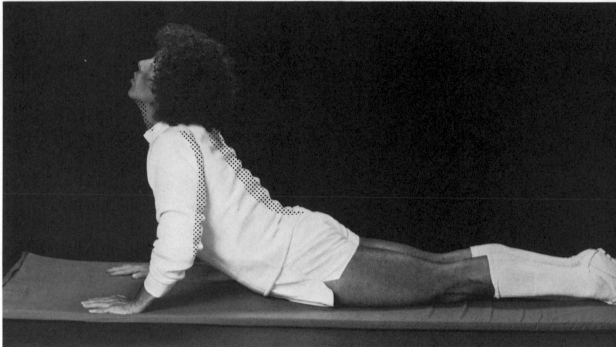

1. Toes are pointed, head is curled back, and palms are flat on the mat with the elbows bent.

2. Pull yourself up and lower yourself down.

B7 Cobra with a Twist

Position: on mat, lying on stomach.

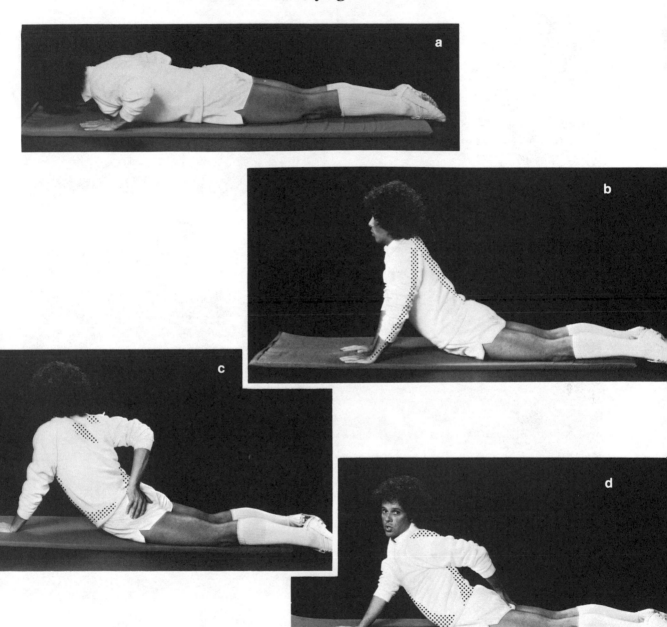

1. Toes are pointed, head is curled back, and palms are flat on the mat with the elbows bent.

2. Take your right arm, put it behind your back, and grab your left hip.

3. Make sure your hips stay on the ground.

4. Alternate sides.

B8 Swan

Position: on mat, lying on stomach.

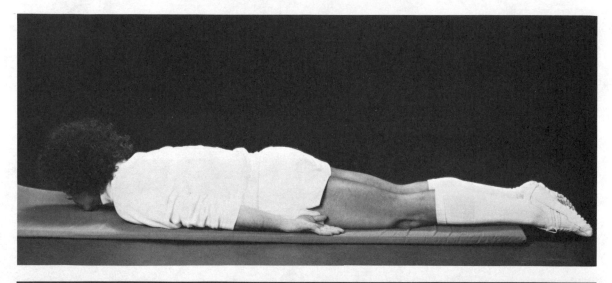

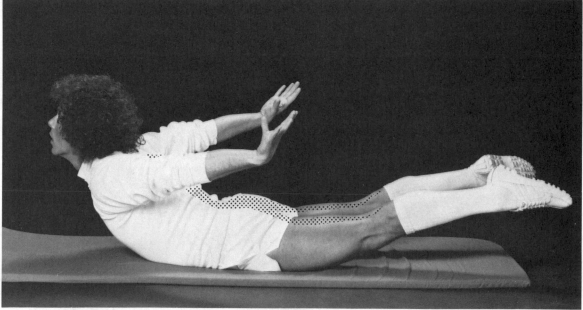

1. With arms at your sides, raise arms slightly into the air, arching your back up.

2. Legs should be straight out behind you and slightly raised into the air, without the knees bent.

B9 Upper Back—Elbow Push-Ups

Position: on mat, on stomach.

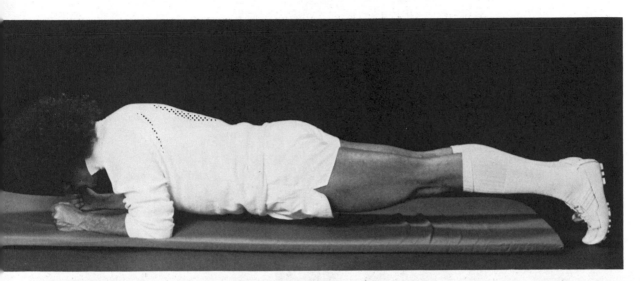

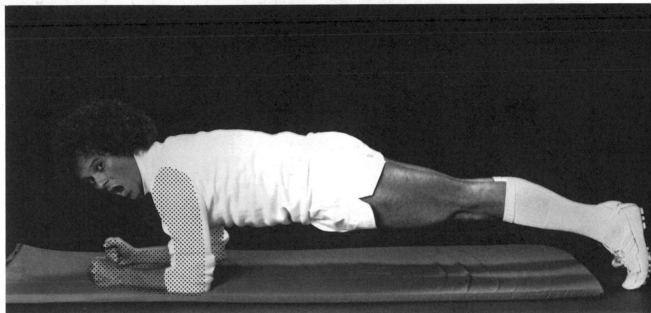

1. Lean on elbows with legs straight out behind you.

2. Push up off the ground on your toes, keeping your body straight.

B10 Upper Back Squeeze

Position: standing, feet slightly apart.

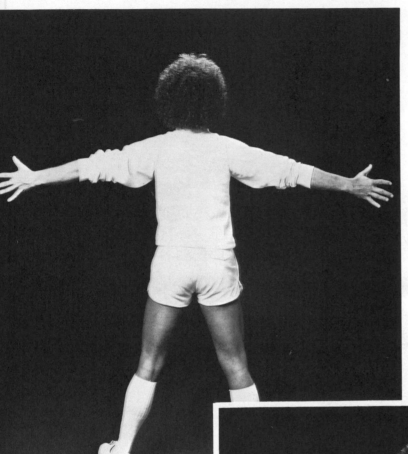

1. Arms are out to the sides at shoulder level.

2. Pull your arms back, squeezing your shoulder blades together, then release.

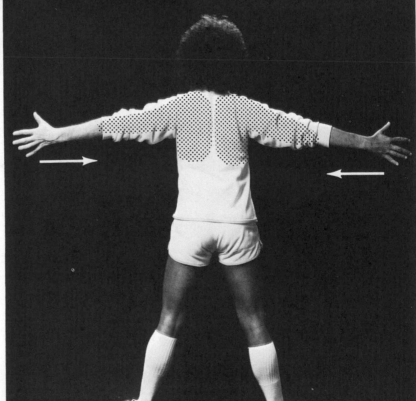

9

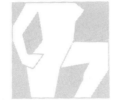

Hips and Thighs

Hip, Hip, Potato Chip

The hips are very much related to the thighs and the buttocks—and often, unfortunately, to the waist—but let's tackle one problem at a time here. I mean, we already know that all parts of the body work so closely together that it's often hard to divide them up into neat little packages, and *hip* seems to be one of those groan words that makes everyone—particularly women—sigh for days.

The most well-known muscle in the hips and the buttocks is the gluteus maximus. (Remember when you were in the fifth grade and you fell into gales of laughter telling someone he gave you a pain in the gluteus maximus?) Well, here it is. There are almost twenty-five muscles (on each side) that make up the hips and the tush area, and if they are not used (and I don't mean to walk and to sit with), they will not be tight—hence the term *flab*—and they will allow fatty deposits to build up beneath them.

The shape of your hips and your buns is not predetermined by your skeleton. Even if everyone in your family has big hips, you can still beat them. (The width of your hips is a skeletal function; their size, however, is not.

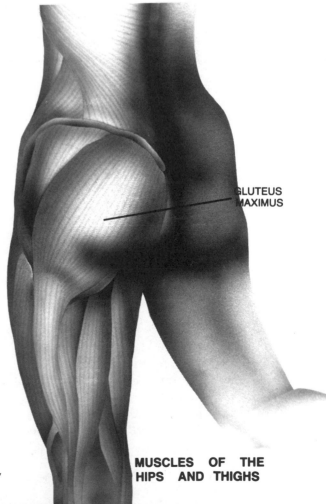

GLUTEUS MAXIMUS

MUSCLES OF THE HIPS AND THIGHS

And, yes, hips can spread with pregnancy.) Unlike some parts of your body, the hips are yours for the molding. Their shape is pretty much determined by exercise.

There are several reasons to keep your hips and your thighs in shape:

1. You don't want anyone to call you bad names that will make you cry.

2. You probably enjoy the simple pleasures, like walking, running, going up stairs, etc.

3. You plan to fit into a bathing suit this summer.

4. You appreciate good posture.

5. You like to prevent backaches before they occur.

6. You don't like the term *middle-age spread*.

7. You don't ever want to have to walk through a door sideways.

8. You want to be able to fit into the bumper cars next time you go to the county fair.

Thigh High Stadium

The muscles attaching the thigh and the pelvis are the groin muscles, and there are several of them, the function of which is to bring the legs together to flex the thighs. Muscles in the calf are responsible for toe pointing and foot stomping. The inside contour of the thigh is the gracilis, which is taken from the Spanish word *gracias*, which is what you say to God if you happen to have a trim, tight gracilis that doesn't bulge or sag. All in

all there are over twenty-five muscles in the legs that give them their shape and make them do their daily work.

Legs are meant to be strong and flexible, not only for getting you from one place to another but for a feeling of body control. How you look in a bathing suit is merely a cosmetic concern, while standing, walking, and even crawling are more basic.

Thigh Control

You'll know it's time to do something about your thighs when:

• your pants don't get over your kneecaps, even though you're already wearing your old maternity pants with the stretched-out elastic and you're not even pregnant.

• you're at a picnic and no one needs to use the table, as lunch is spread across your lap and there's room for everything.

• your child thinks that in the story "Little Red Ridinghood" the little girl looks up at the wolf in grandmother's clothing and says, "Grandmother, what big thighs you have."

• you're dressed in your favorite bathing

suit and notice that your thighs bulge out enough to form a shelf on which to stand a canned soft drink. Furthermore, the shelf doesn't even wobble.

• your child reaches for your skirt to cling to and instead gets a handful of your thigh— and it doesn't even hurt you.

• you buy a skirt that is two sizes too big in order to accommodate your hips and then have to ask the store to alter only the bottom part of the skirt by taking some of the extra fullness from around your knees.

• you're standing upright with your legs together and you can start a fire from the friction caused by your thighs meeting.

Why My Thigh? Oh, Sigh!

There's a very good reason why you have chubby thighs. No, it has nothing to do with your metabolism—or your thyroid. It's an honest to goodness, no bull reason that very few people—even people with heavy thighs—ever learn. You just don't happen to use your thigh muscles that often.

The thigh muscles work along with several other muscles in that general neighborhood—you know them all—the abdominals, the buttocks, the hips, and the calves. The jobs the thigh muscles do—extending and distending the lower leg, rotating to and fro, and doing the hootchy-kootchy—just aren't normal actions in a person's day. Sure, you may walk up and down a lot of stairs, but never enough to keep your thigh muscles in shape.

The only way to keep your thigh muscles firm is to actually exercise them! Daily routine—unless you are an acrobat—just doesn't give them the workout they need.

Cottage Cheese Thighs

Do you suffer from lumps and bumps of dimply cottage cheese that someone accidentally stuffed between the skin in your thighs and the muscles? The beauty experts are big on calling this cellulite and advocating all kinds of treatments (mostly expensive) to wrap, sweat, exercise, or starve the little critters away.

Well, folks, I've got big news for you.

There's no such thing as cellulite.

Ask any doctor. (I did.)

There is such a thing as fat. Fat has a tendency to build up in certain parts of the body, because they are more accessible than other parts. The thighs are one of these areas, particularly in women. (On men it's the love handles.) In people who have loose, weak muscles and no tone in their legs, the fat cells run crazy and build very modern structures. There are no zoning laws, because the only outward dimension they have to deal with is your skin. So the reason the fat looks lumpy and bumpy is because it has spread out into suburbs, built a few high rises here and there, and run all over your interior map without an architect. Since the fat cells are everywhere, it's hard to exercise them out. Exercise will firm up the muscle underneath but will not kill fat cells. (Nothing kills fat cells.)

Can you CURE cottage cheese thighs?

Nope. (Forget about that herbal wrap treatment you've been saving for.)

Can you PREVENT cottage cheese thighs?

Yes, you can.

You can prevent those ripples and dimples from appearing by eating properly and by keeping your legs in such good form that there is no room for the fat cells to accumulate and to do their ugly damage.

By the way, so-called cellulite affects thin people as well as overweighters. Anyone who is physically out of shape and has not built up strong leg muscles will suffer. You can have the figure of a Playboy bunny and still have cottage cheese thighs—so take care to prevent them with serious exercise and by eating properly.

HT1 Cat Stretches

Position: on mat, on hands and knees.

1. Knees are apart, palms are flat on the ground.

2. Lower your head, inhale, arch your back, raise your head, and exhale, then lower your head, inhale, etc.

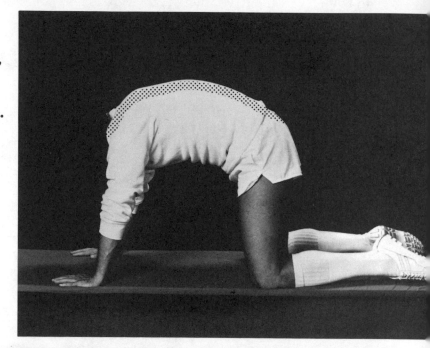

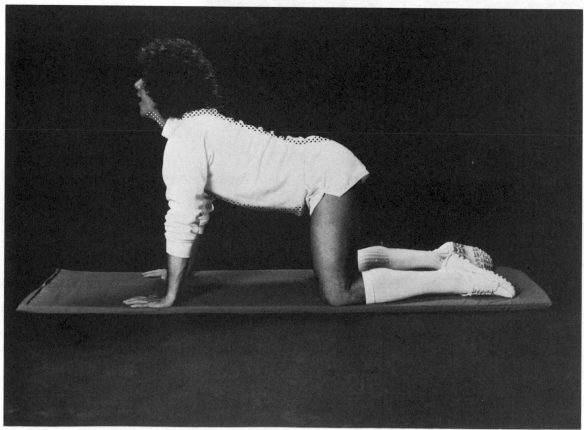

HT2 Knee to Chest

Position: on mat, on hands and knees.

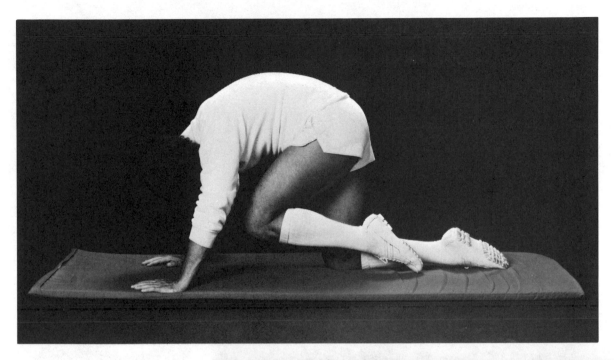

1. Keeping left leg slightly bent, bring leg in to your nose, then kick it back.

2. Alternate sides.

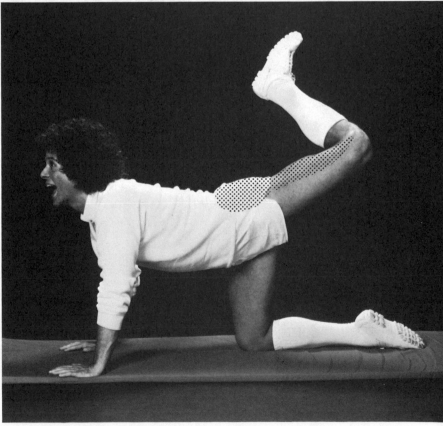

HT3 Donkey Kick

Position: on mat, on hands and knees.

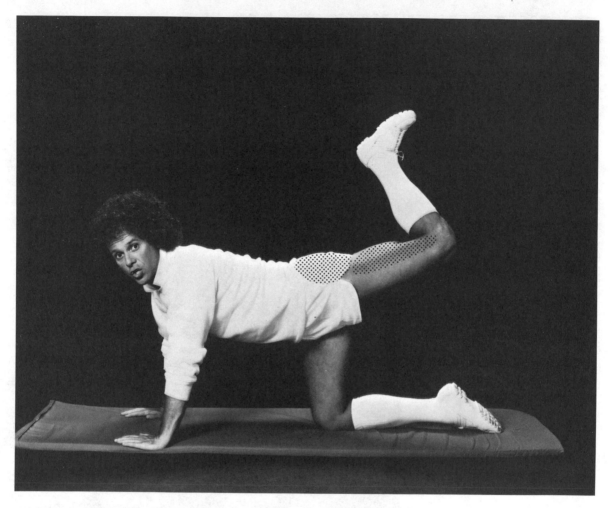

1. **Keeping left leg slightly bent, lift the leg from the hip, not the knee.**

2. **Keep foot flexed.**

3. **Alternate sides.**

HT4 *Kicks to the Back*

Position: on mat, on hands and knees.

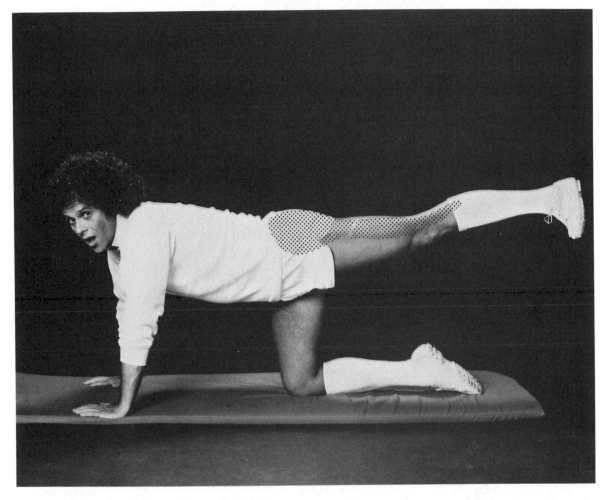

1. Keeping left leg straight out behind you, flex foot and lift. (Don't drop your knee.)

2. Alternate sides.

HT5 Kicks to the Side

Position: on mat, on hands and knees.

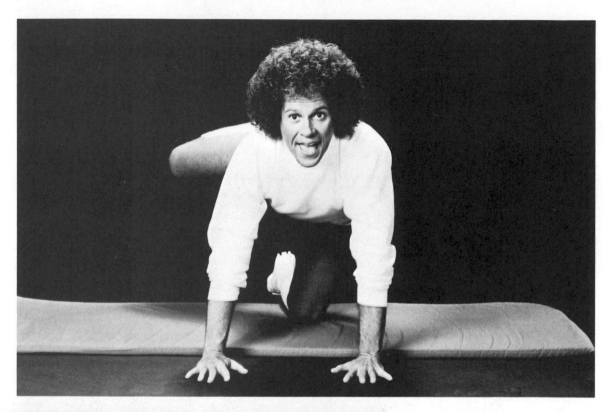

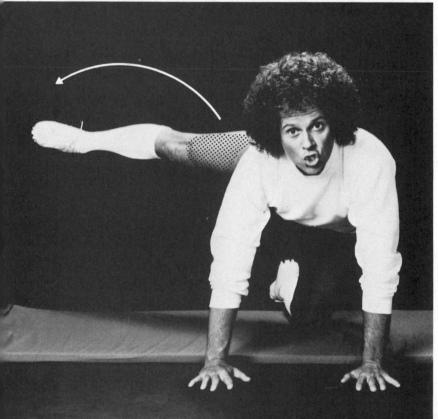

1. Keeping right leg slightly bent and foot flexed, kick to the side.

2. Alternate sides.

3. You should also feel this in your tush!

HT6 Knee to Chest and Side

Position: on mat, on hands and knees.

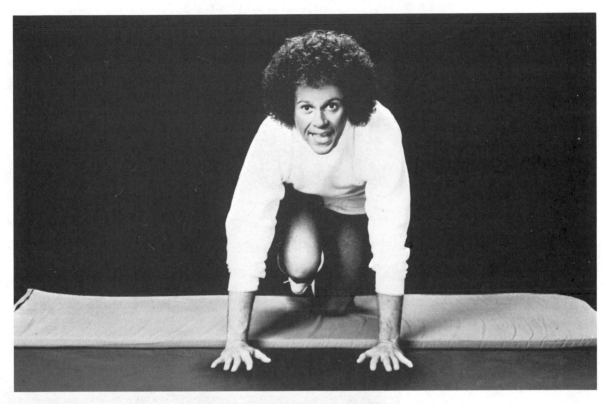

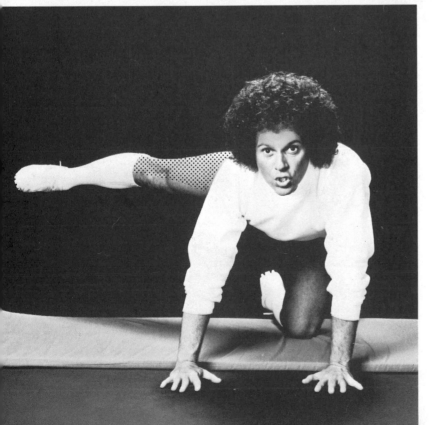

1. **Bring right knee in to chest, then kick it out to the side.**

2. **Alternate sides.**

3. **You should also feel this in your tush.**

HT7 Doggy Lifts

Position: on mat, on hands and knees.

1. Keeping right leg bent, lift it to the side, then put it down.

2. Alternate sides.

3. You should also feel this in your tush.

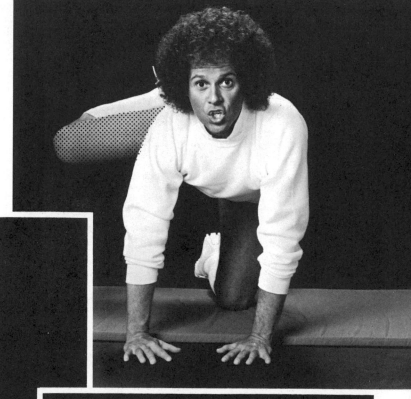

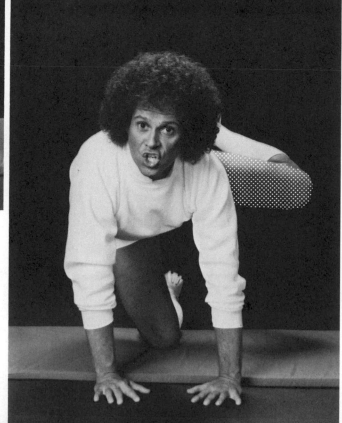

HT8 Doggy Lift Holds

Position: on mat, on hands and knees.

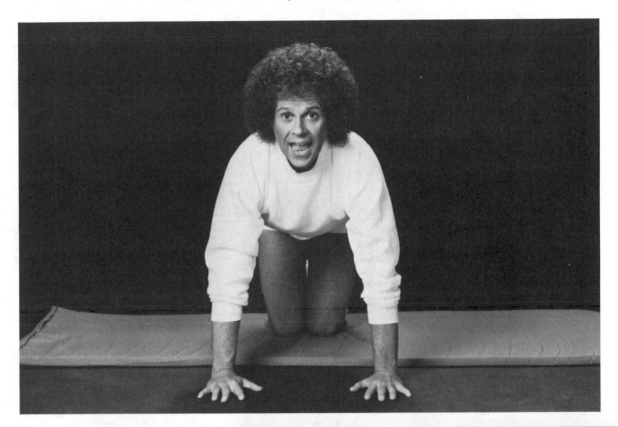

1. Keeping right leg bent, lift it to the side as high as you can, then bring it down—but hold it up as long as you can. (Boy, will you feel this in your tush!)

2. Alternate sides.

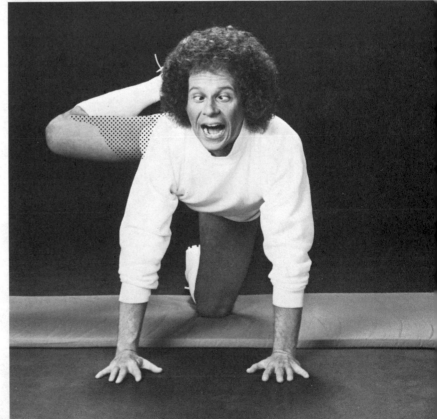

HT9 Doggy Lift Kicks

Position: on mat, on hands and knees.

1. Keeping right leg bent, lift it to the side, then kick it out, then bring it down.

2. Alternate sides.

3. You should also feel this in your tush.

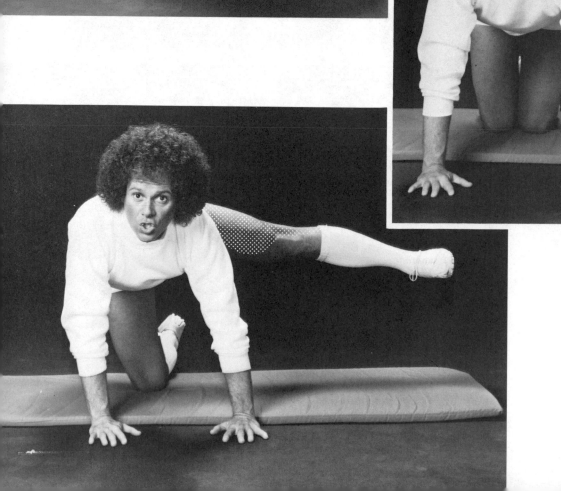

HT10 Knee to Shoulder Twists

Position: on mat, on hands and knees.

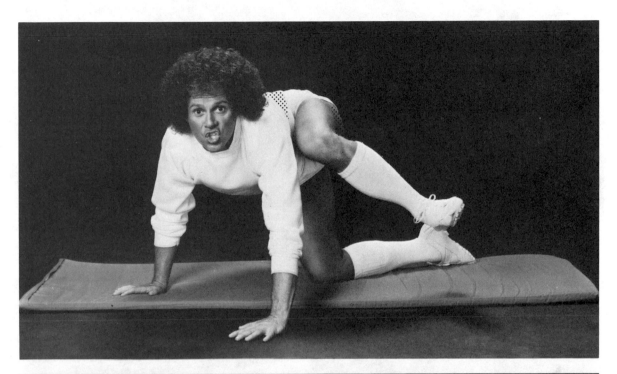

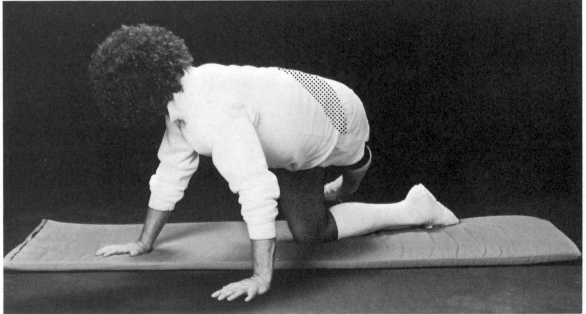

1. Raise left leg with bent knee and bring it to your left shoulder.

2. Bring same leg straight back and across to your right side while looking over your right shoulder. (Try to look for your toes.)

3. Alternate sides.

HT11 Straight Leg Twists

Position: on mat, on hands and knees.

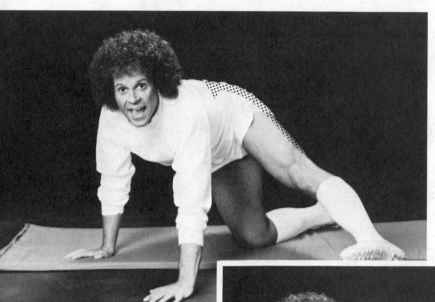

1. Bring left leg forward with foot flexed, then smoothly bring same leg back and over to your right side while looking over your right shoulder.

2. Make sure back leg is well stretched.

3. Alternate sides.

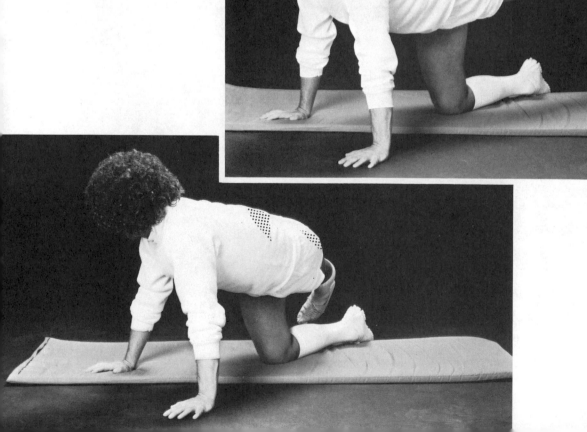

HT12 Hip Rolls

Position: on mat, on hands and knees.

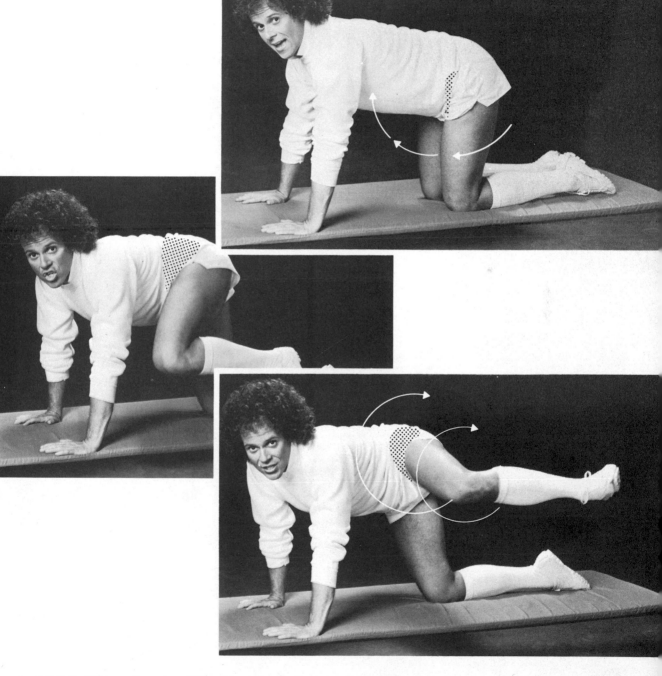

1. With left knee bent, roll leg in a circle forward, then back.

2. Alternate sides.

HT13 Half Circle Rotations

Position: on mat, on hands and knees.

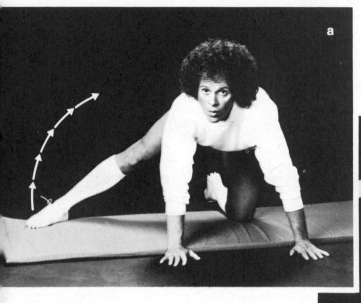

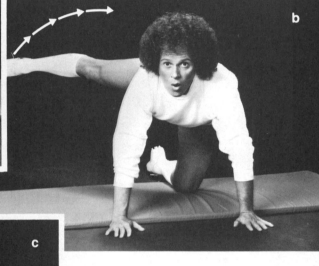

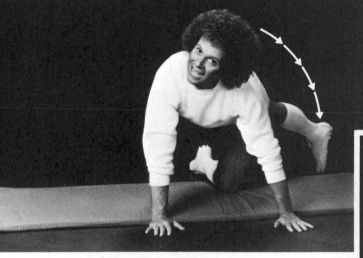

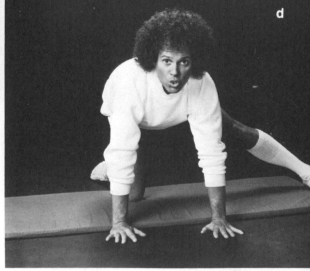

1. **With right leg straight out to the side, lift it up and over to the other side.**

2. **Point your foot.**

3. **Alternate sides.**

4. **You should feel this in your tush.**

HT14 Knee Waves

Position: sitting on knees on mat.

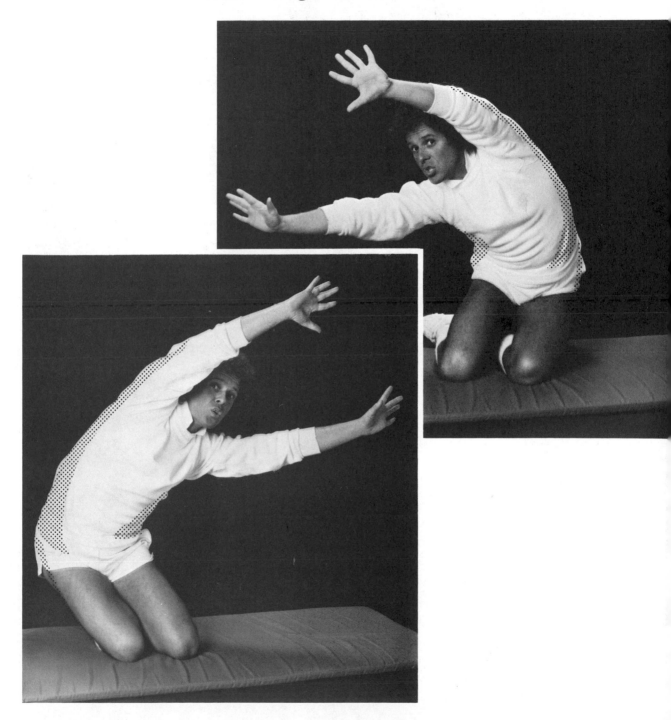

1. **Leaning to the left, raise arms overhead and wave to the right.**

2. **Leaning to the right, raise arms overhead and wave to the left.**

3. **Alternate sides.**

HT15 Praise the Lords

Position: sitting on knees on mat.

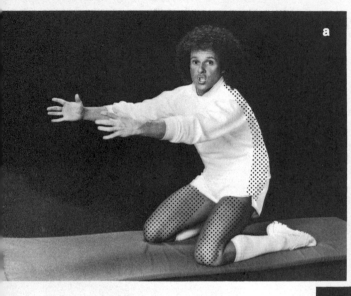

1. Sit back on your heels,
raise yourself up, and lower
yourself down.

2. Don't sit all the way back.

3. At the same time move
arms backward and
forward with palms facing
down.

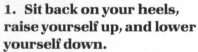

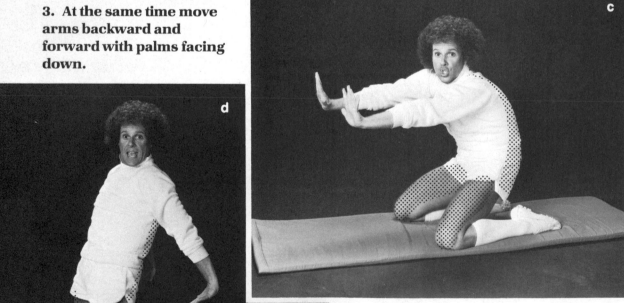

HT16 Hip Flips

Position: on mat, sitting on buns.

1. Knees are bent, legs are apart.

2. As you bring your left knee over to your right side, stretch your arms over to your left side.

3. Keep your back straight and your chest forward.

4. Alternate sides.

5. You should feel this in your upper back, too.

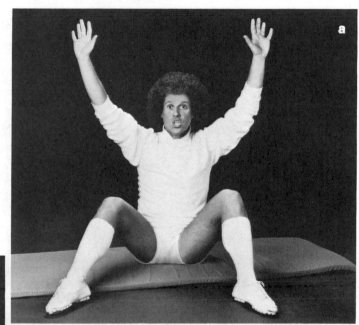

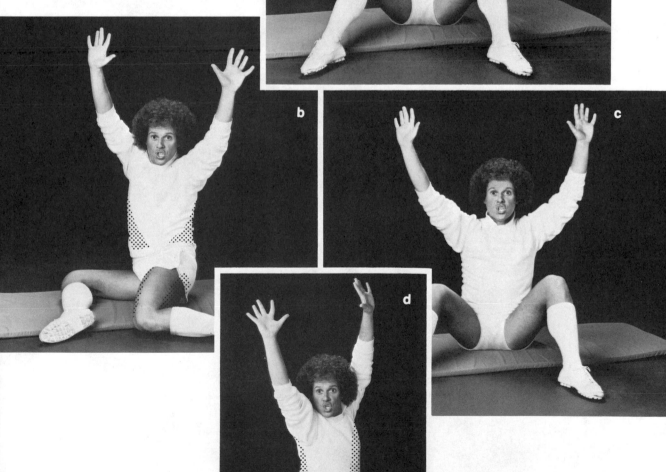

HT17 Tootsie Rolls

Position: on mat, sitting up.

1. Legs are straight out in front of you.

2. Roll your hips to the left, then roll to the right in a continuous motion. Swing your arms in the opposite direction to which you are rolling.

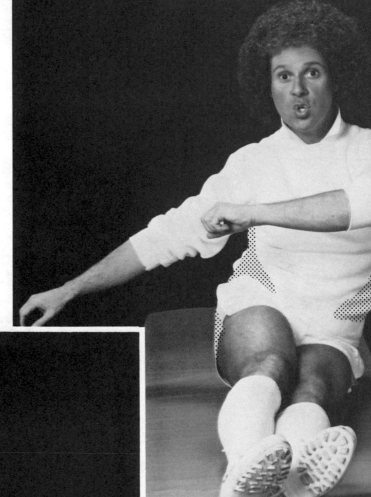

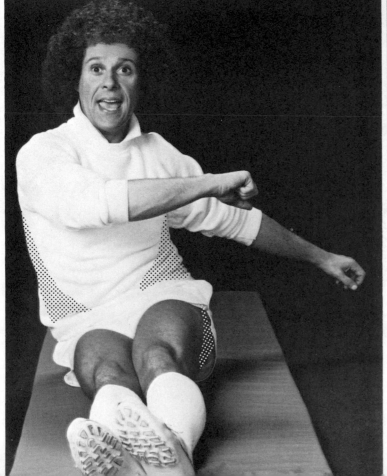

HT18 Knee over Tootsie Rolls

Position: on mat, sitting up.

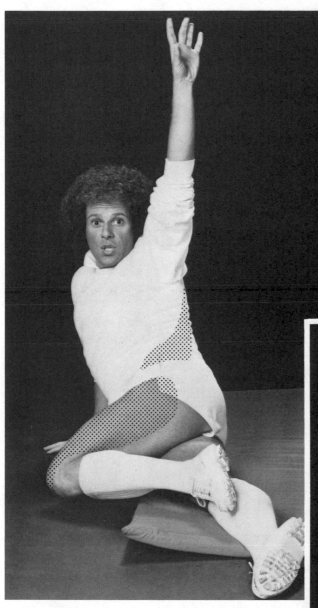

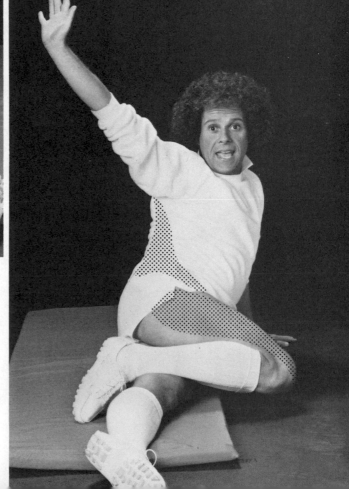

1. Legs are straight out in front of you.

2. Bending your left knee, roll your hips to the right and cross your left knee over your right leg. Use your arms for balance.

3. Alternate sides.

HT19 Tootsie Pops

Position: on mat, sitting up.

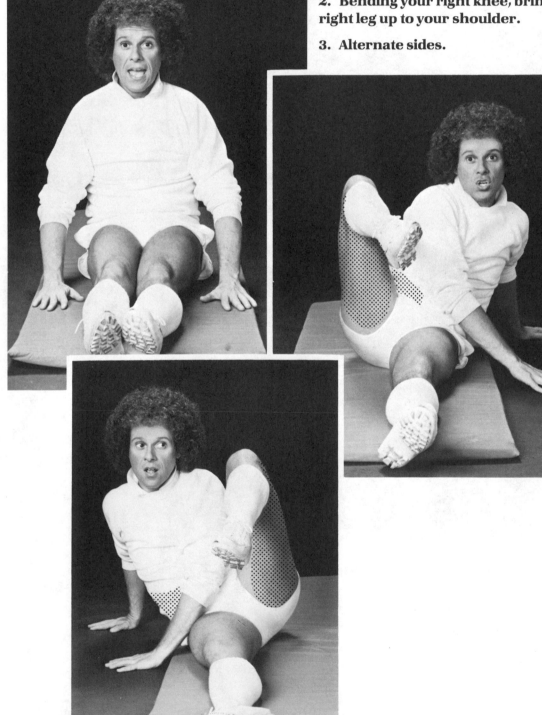

1. Legs are straight out in front of you.

2. Bending your right knee, bring your right leg up to your shoulder.

3. Alternate sides.

HT20 *Thigh Squeezes*

Position: on mat, sitting with knees bent and feet on floor.
Arms are to the side with weight on your palms.

1. **Raise your buns into the air, then move your knees in and out.**

2. **Squeeze for in, release for out.**

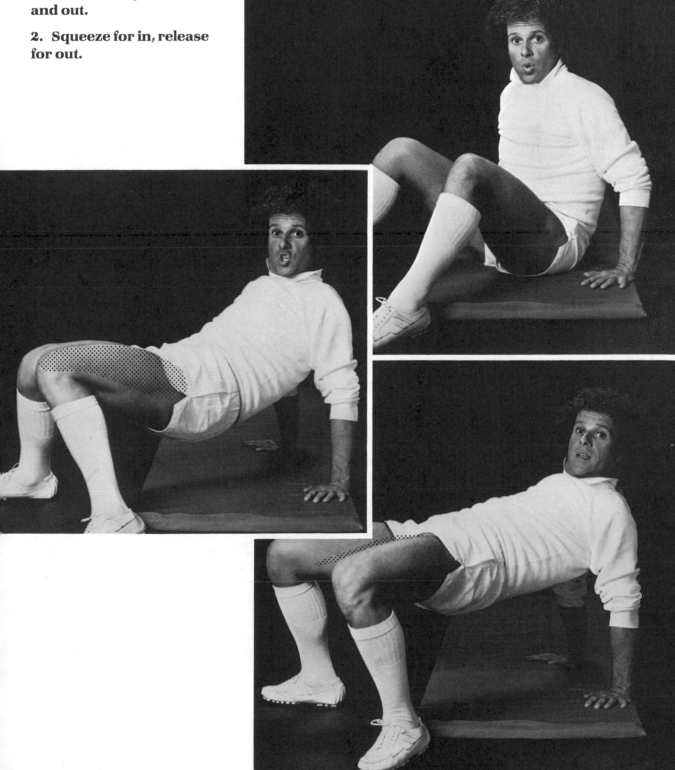

10

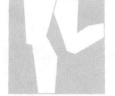

Legs and Calves

Leg Call

Quick, check the kind of legs you have:

☐ bird
☐ dinosaur
☐ chicken
☐ mosquito.

Well, whatever type it is, I have good news for you. Exercise can make it better. The only part of your legs that the skeleton determines is how tall or how short they are. Shapeliness is all a matter of exercise (unless you are bowlegged or knock-kneed). So the rest is up to you.

If the only thing you depend on your legs for is getting to the 7-Eleven at 4:00 A.M., you are indeed in bad shape. If the only thing you think of when I say leg is (A) turkey legs, (B) frogs' legs, or (C) leg of lamb, you are in bad shape. But, when I say leg, and you think (A) lifts, (B) circles, and (C) kicks, you're warming up.

After all, your legs and calves are very important not only to your figure but to your locomotion. Legs are the most robust parts of the body. The bones of the legs are connected to the hips by the pelvic girdle. The pelvic girdle helps shift the weight of the upper body to the lower limbs—your legs—since the main function of the legs is to support your weight.

The leg is made up of three main bones, much like an arm, although legs bear so much more weight than arms that they are thicker and sturdier. (At least mine are.) The gluteus maximus, which comprises the buns and part of the thigh, is one of the strongest muscles in your whole body. The main muscles of the calves are the gastrocnemius and the soleus, both of which are attached at the heel by the Achilles tendon. The fronts of the calves are generally called the shins.

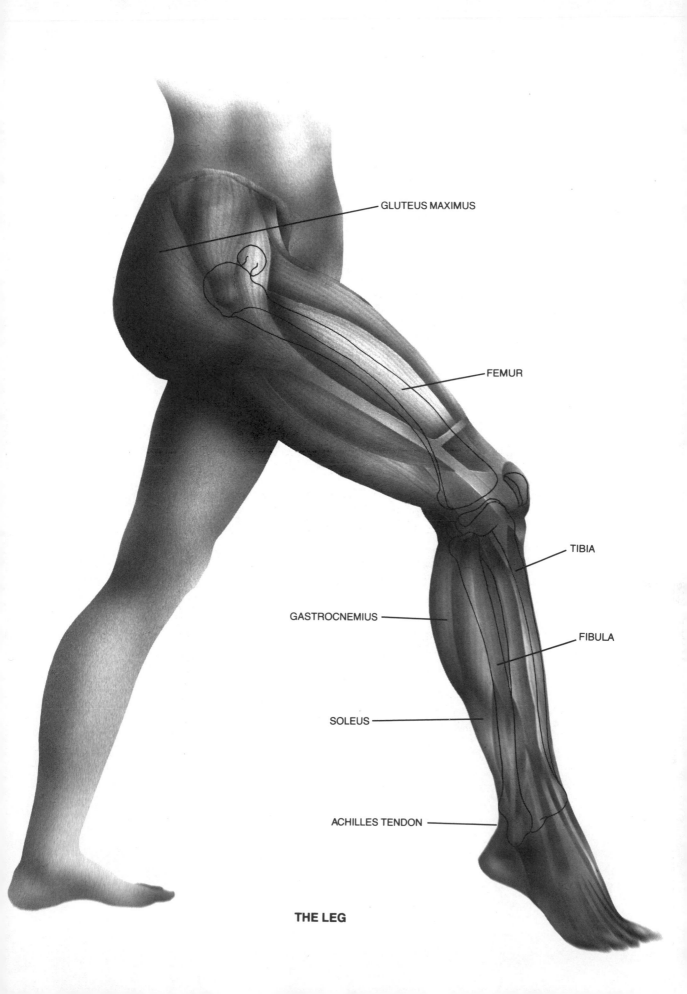

GLUTEUS MAXIMUS

FEMUR

TIBIA

GASTROCNEMIUS

FIBULA

SOLEUS

ACHILLES TENDON

THE LEG

Tired Legs

That crummy feeling of throbbing, tired legs usually comes from the accumulation of lactic acid in the muscles. Since the blood can get only a certain amount of oxygen to your muscles at one given time, and your muscles continue working (even while you're walking long distances or shopping too much) without oxygen, lactic acid is produced. And that's how you get muscle cramps and pains. Relax the muscles for a while so they are not forced to contract, and the blood will make the lactic acid go bye-bye, and you will feel better. You can help prevent the pains before you get them by avoiding some of these situations:

- walking barefoot on pavement, concrete, pebbles, or gravel
- wearing shoes that are not fitted properly or boots that are too tight for exercise
- exercising on wooden or concrete floors without a mat—especially when you are jumping and putting weight down on your legs (That's how you get what is called shin-splints.)
- bad posture habits and poor body alignment (Straighten it out!)
- a job that requires being on your feet all day—especially if you are in high heels.

The Joe Namath Honorary Knee Knewsletter

The knee is the largest joint in the body. It can be affected by tension, bad posture, high heels, poorly fitted shoes, hard surfaces, strenuous activities, and being tackled. Overweighters increase the strain on their knees because they are forcing extra weight to be borne by the joints. (Yes, there's even something called housemaid's knee—an inflammation of the joint that you can get from too much kneeling. AND there's something called clergyman's knee, which comes from kneeling in a more upright position.) The knee can suffer a direct bruise, or fluid can accumulate in the joint and make you miserable. You can also break the patella (kneecap), which is extremely painful.

Exercise cannot actually strengthen the knees, so they remain vulnerable and in need of care.

L1 Knee to Chest

Position: on mat, lying on side.

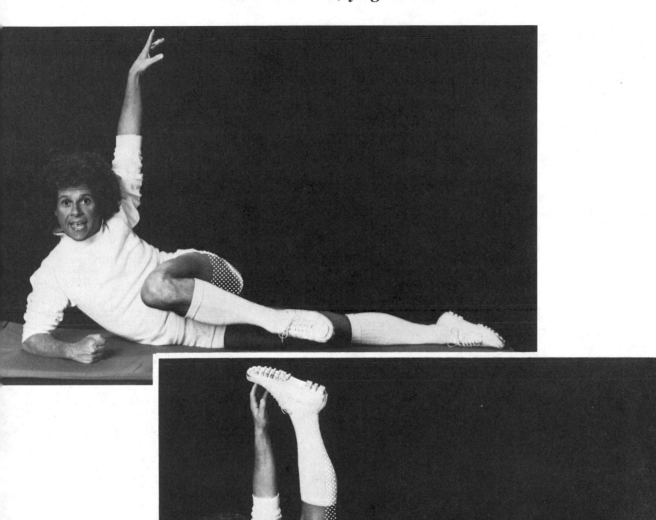

1. **Support yourself on your right elbow.**

2. **Bring your left knee into your chest, straighten your leg out, then lift it straight up.**

3. **Alternate sides.**

L2 Knee to Shoulder

Position: on mat, lying on side.

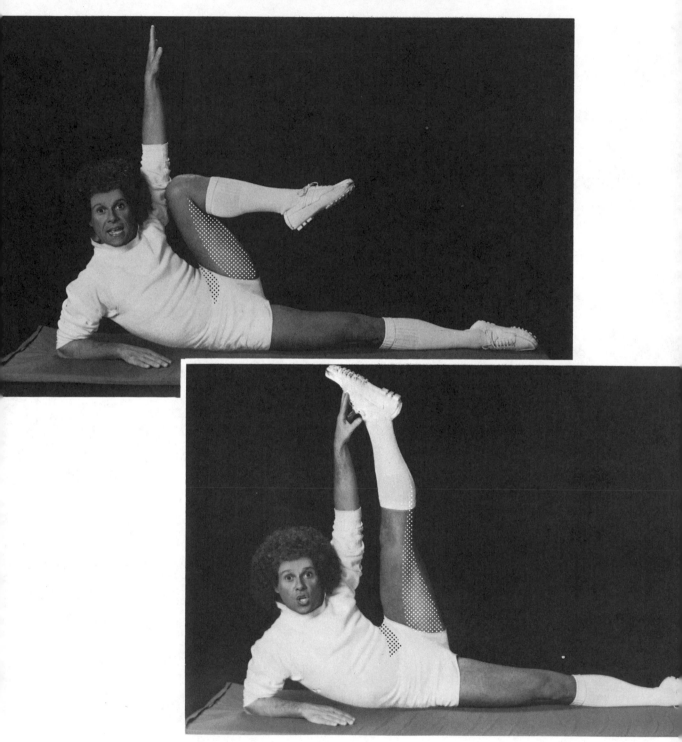

1. **Support yourself on your right elbow.**

2. **Bring your left knee up to your shoulder, then extend your leg straight up.**

3. **Alternate sides.**

L3 Side Leg Lifts

Position: on mat, lying on side, supported by one elbow.

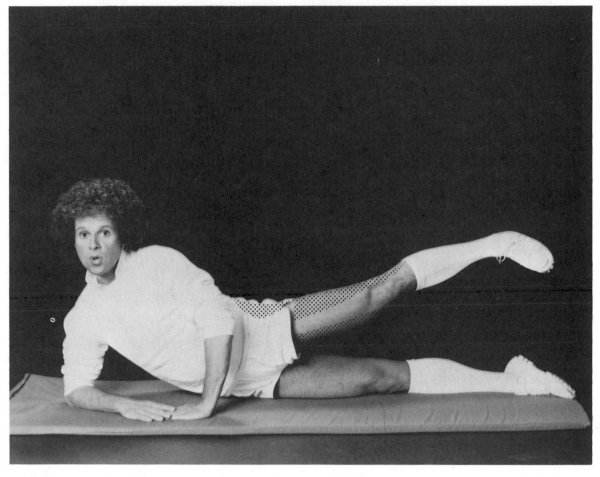

1. Keep your chest up and your abdomen in.

2. Lift left leg up while flexed at ankle so heel is higher than toes. Keep hip forward, and don't worry about raising it up too high—its impossible!

3. Alternate sides.

L4 *Side Leg Circles*

Position: on mat, lying on side, supported by elbow and hand.

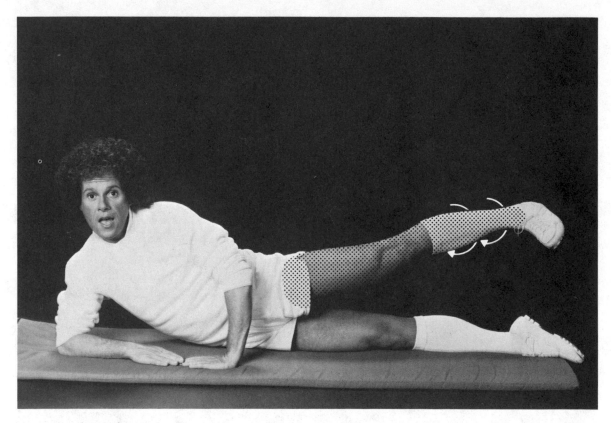

1. Lift left leg halfway up and circle around to the front, then to the back.

2. Alternate sides.

L5 Front Leg Minilifts

Position: on mat, lying on side, supported by elbow and hand.

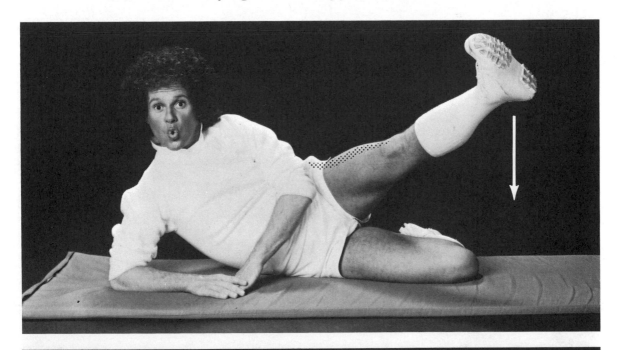

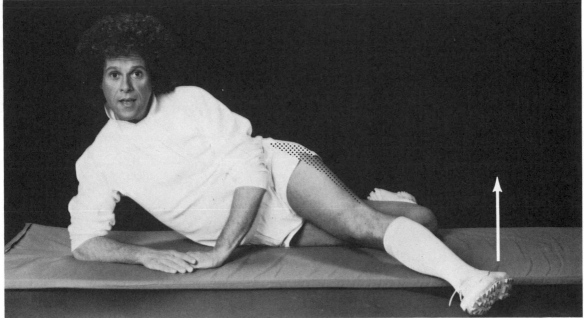

1. Lying on right side, bend right knee and push leg back.

2. Keep upper (left) leg straight, then tilt it slightly forward with ankle flexed.

3. In this position do leg lifts without throwing your weight backward or forward too much.

4. Alternate sides.

L6 Circles Forward

Position: on mat, lying on side, supported by elbow and hand.

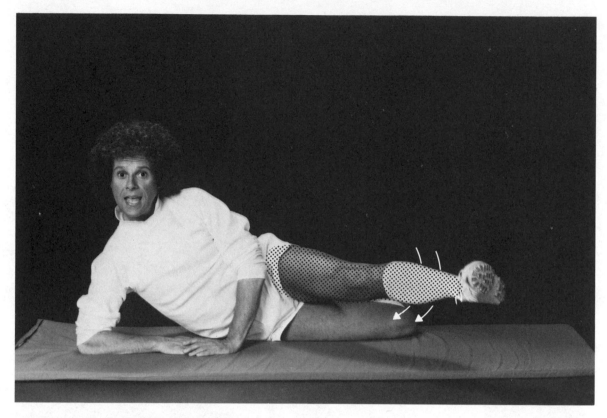

1. **Lying on right side, bend right knee and push leg back.**

2. **Keep left leg straight, then tilt left leg and hip slightly forward with ankle flexed.**

3. **Circle left leg around to the front, then to the back.**

4. **Alternate sides.**

L7 Complete Front Leg Lifts

Position: on mat, lying on side, supported by elbow and hand.

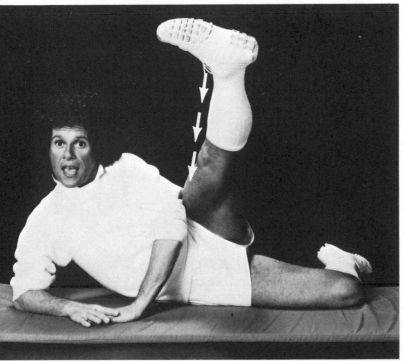

1. **Lying on right side, bend right knee and push leg back.**

2. **Keep left leg straight, move it forward, then raise and lower it from a position a few inches above the floor.**

3. **DON'T sit forward or lie back. Keep body aligned.**

4. **Alternate sides.**

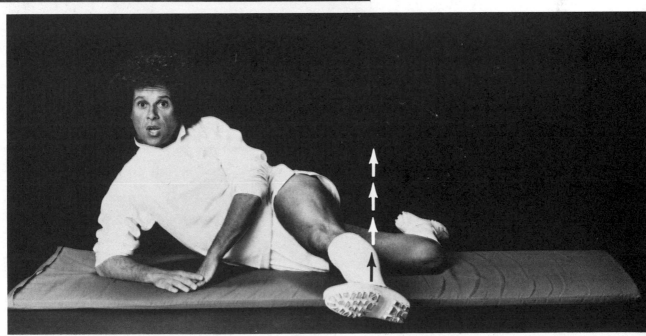

L8 Complete Leg Stretches

Position: on mat, lying on side, supported by elbow and hand.

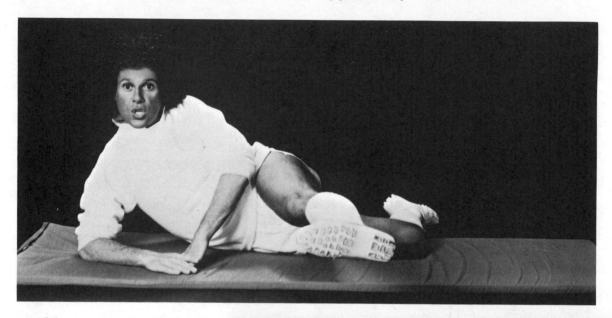

1. This exercise is similar to Complete Front Leg Lift, but use your left arm to stretch your left leg as far over as possible.

2. You push that top leg with your hand to really get the stretch moving and to make life a little easier.

3. Repeat stretches, then alternate sides.

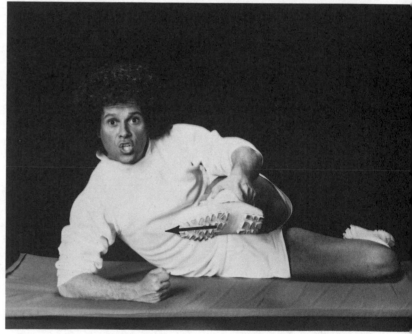

L9 Inner Thigh Lifts

Position: on mat, lying on side, supported by elbow and hand.

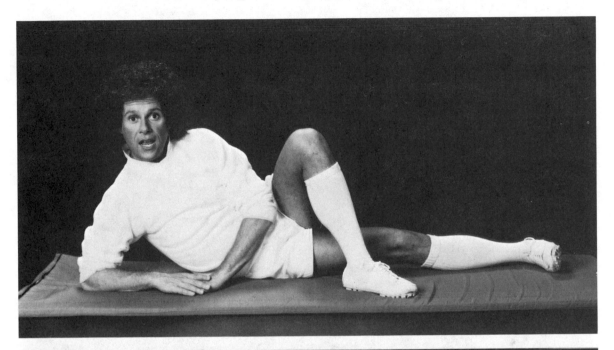

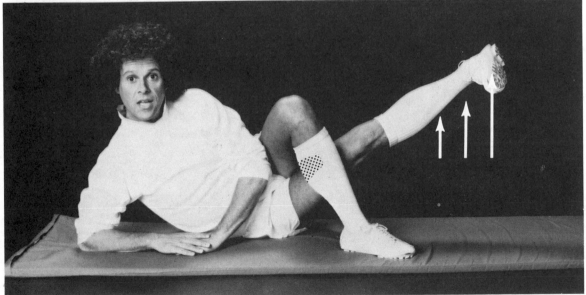

1. **Cross left leg over right and bend your knee, forming an inverted V.**

2. **Lift bottom leg.**

3. **Alternate sides.**

L10 Advanced Inner Thighs

Position: on mat, lying on side, supported by elbow and hand.

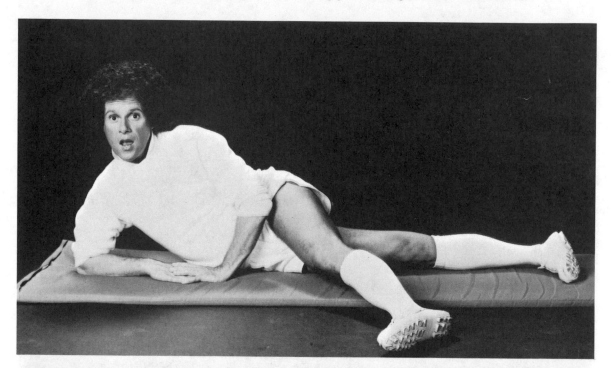

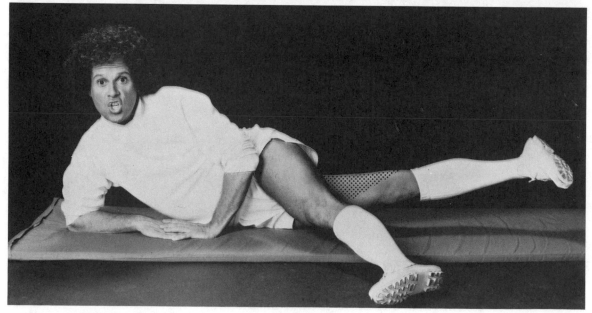

1. **Cross straight left leg over right. Lift bottom leg.**

2. **Flex and point as you lift.**

3. **Alternate sides.**

L11 Circles Down Under

Position: on mat, lying on side, supported by elbow and hand.

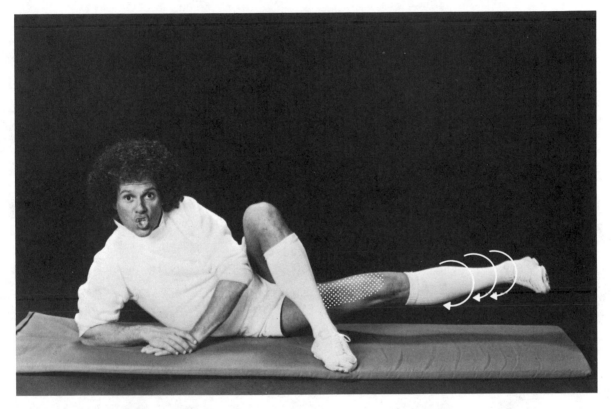

1. Cross left leg over right and bend your left leg at knee, forming an inverted V.

2. Lift bottom leg and circle it forward.

3. Alternate sides.

4. You should feel this in your inner thighs.

L12 Advanced Circles Down Under

Position: on mat, lying on side, supported by elbow and hand.

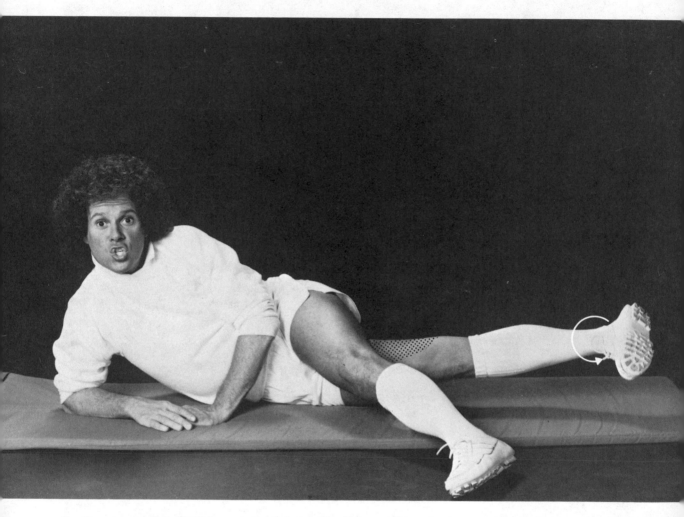

1. **Cross straight left leg over right. Raise lower leg and make small forward circles with foot flexed.**

2. **Alternate sides.**

L13 Inner Thighs on Back *(Not for Overweighters!)*

Position: on mat, lying on back.

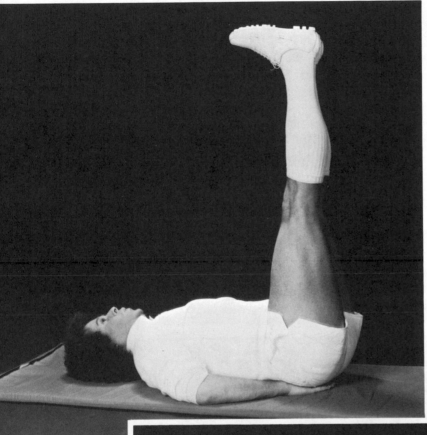

1. Place hands under buttocks and keep shoulders on the ground.

2. Lift legs straight up into the air and flex feet.

3. Open and close legs.

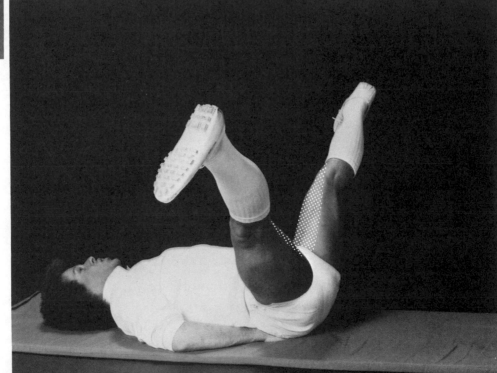

L14 Sitting Inner Thighs

Position: on mat, sitting up straight.

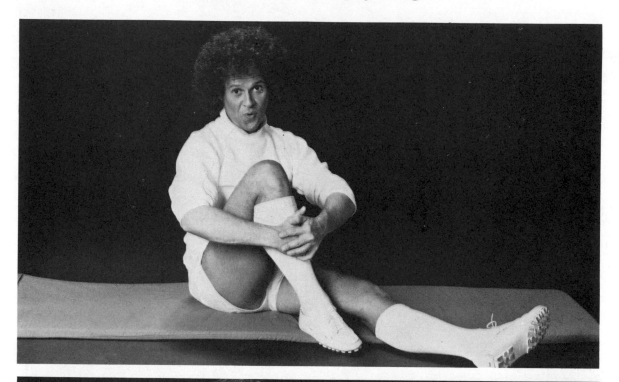

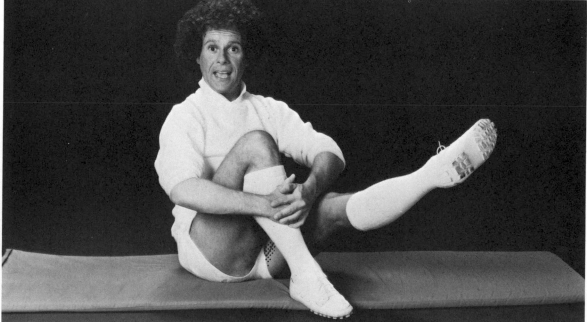

1. **Bend one knee and keep the other leg straight.**

2. **Lift straight leg as high as you can with foot flexed.**

3. **Alternate sides.**

L15 Side Swipes

Position: on mat, sitting up very straight.

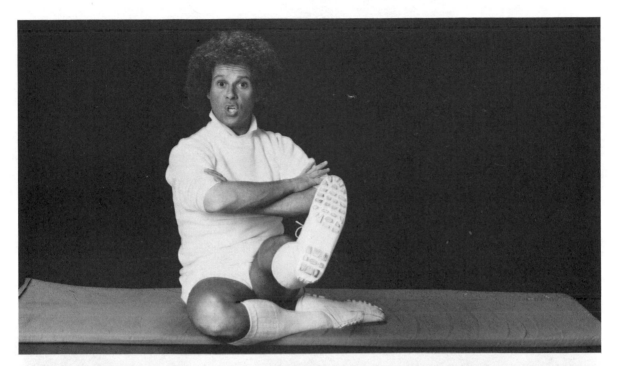

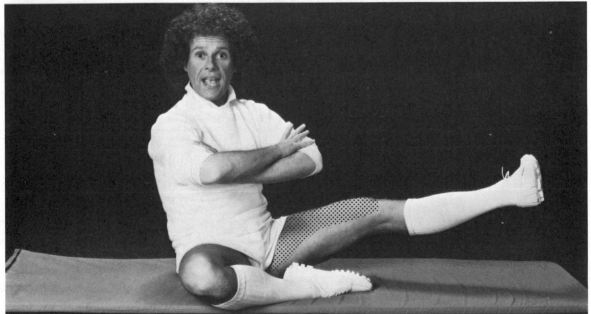

1. **Bend right knee and bring heel in toward your body.**

2. **Lift left leg straight out and as high as you can with foot flexed, then move out to the left.**

3. **Alternate sides.**

L16 Heel Lifts

Position: on mat, standing with feet apart.

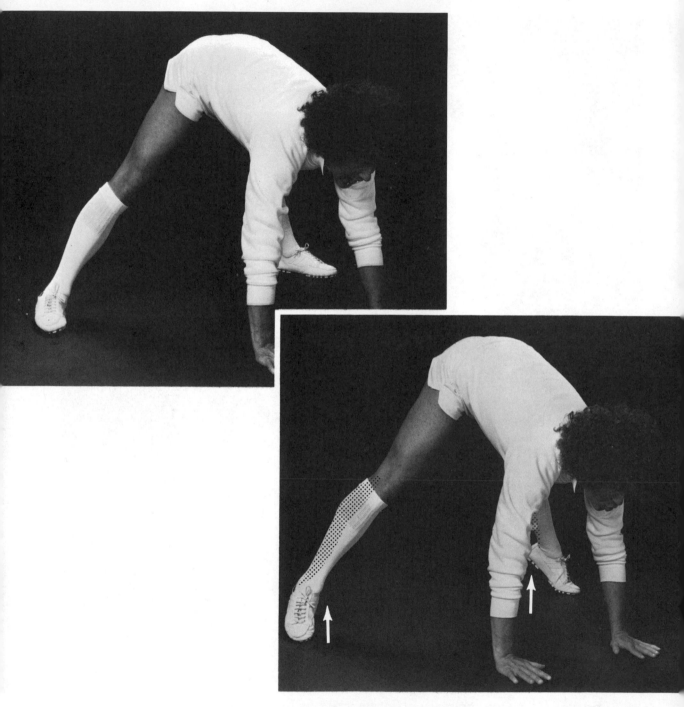

1. Bend over and place palms down on floor in front of you.

2. Lift heels off the ground.

L17 Toe Lifts

Position: on mat, standing.

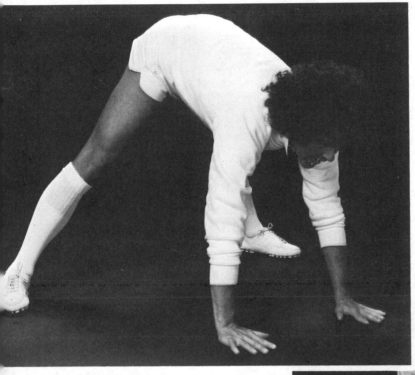

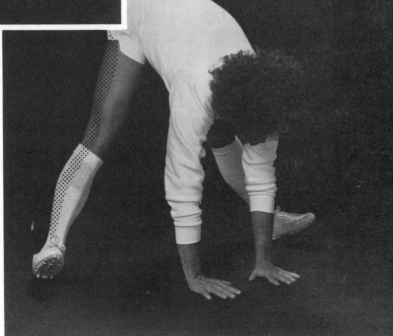

1. Bend over and place palms down on floor in front of you. Walk palms backward, lifting from the waist.

2. Raise your toes up as far as you can while balancing on your heels.

L18 Heel Walks

Position: on mat, standing.

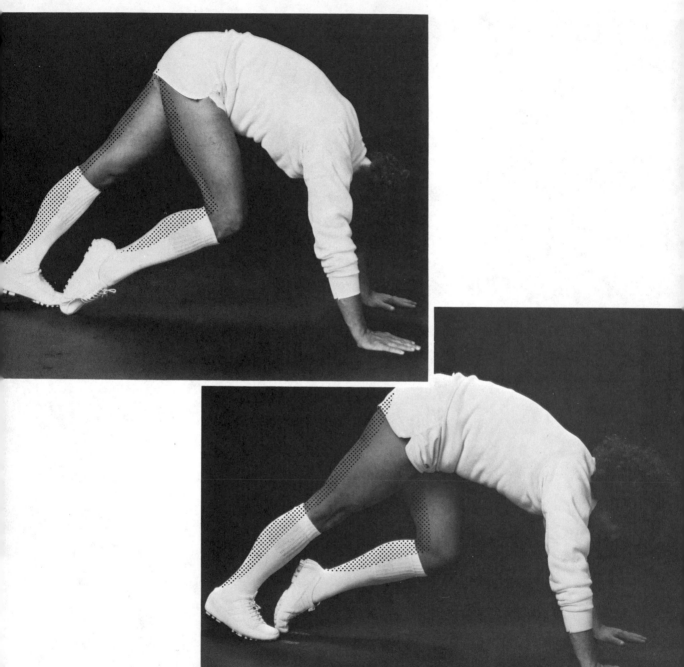

1. Bend over with palms on floor and legs out behind you.

2. Move heels up and down as you pretend to walk up a flight of stairs. (What a funny way to walk up stairs!)

L19 Side Lunges

Position: on mat, standing.

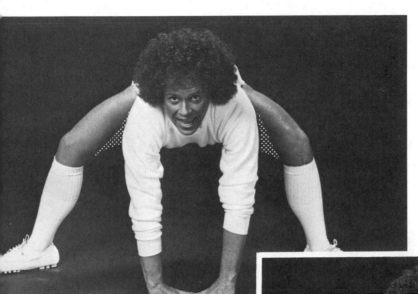

1. **Facing forward, move feet wide apart.**

2. **Place palms down on the floor in the center.**

3. **Keeping your buns in the air, lean to the right, bending the right knee, but keep the left leg straight.**

4. **Alternate sides.**

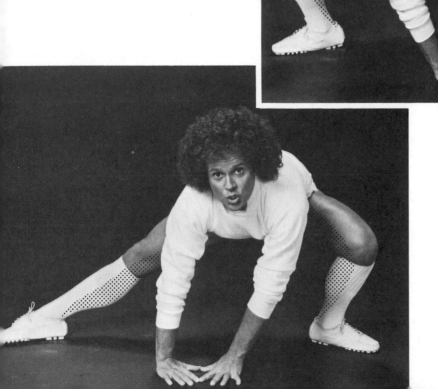

L20 Profile Lunge Hold

Position: on mat, standing.

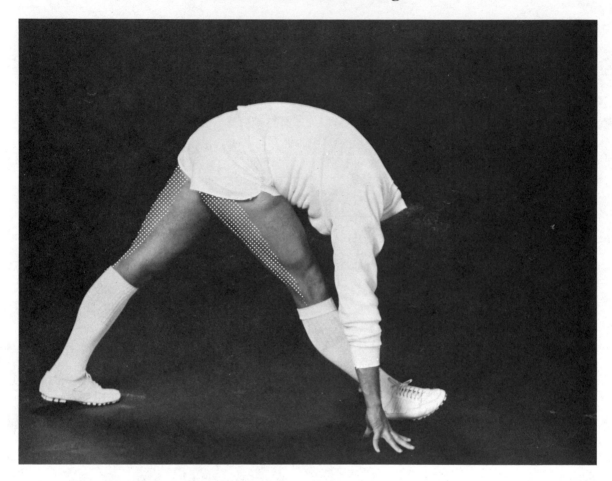

1. Facing forward, move feet wide apart.

2. Place palms down on floor.

3. Keeping both legs straight, lean to the right and hold,
then lean to the left and hold.

L21 *Profile Lunge Down*

Position: on mat, standing.

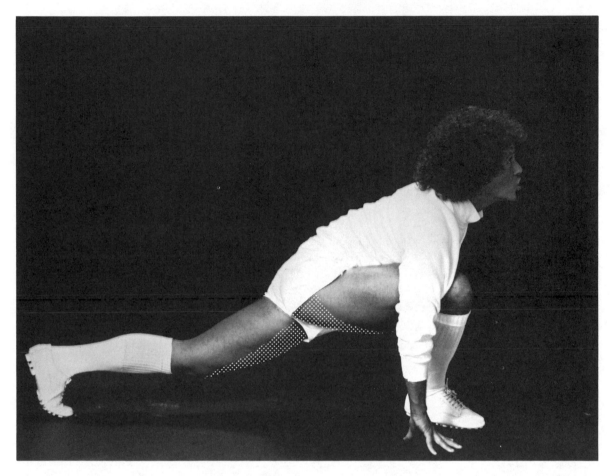

1. **Facing forward, move feet wide apart.**

2. **Place palms down on floor.**

3. **Turn to the right side, bend right leg, and lunge down, keeping left leg straight out behind you.**

4. **Alternate sides.**

L22 Lunge Up and Down

Position: on mat, standing.

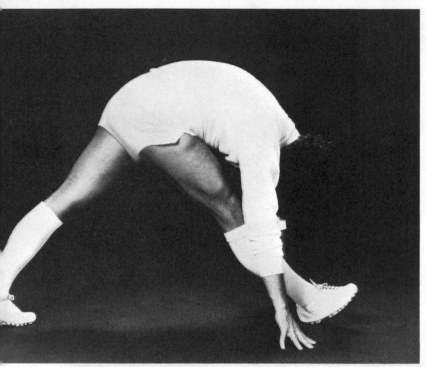

1. **Bend over, feet wide apart, with fingers pressed to floor and head down.**

2. **Bend right leg, lunge forward, then rock back.**

3. **Alternate sides.**

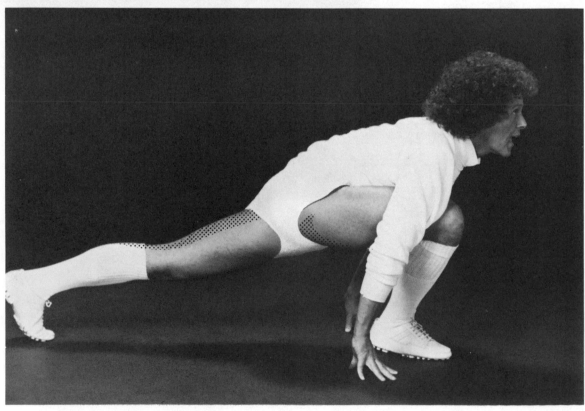

L23 Squats

Position: on mat, standing.

1. Place feet together, balancing on toes.

2. Squat down.

3. Keep fingers pressed to the floor, raise buns, bring heels down, then stand up.

4. Squat, stand, squat, etc.

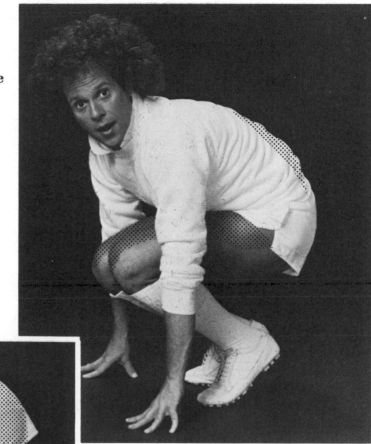

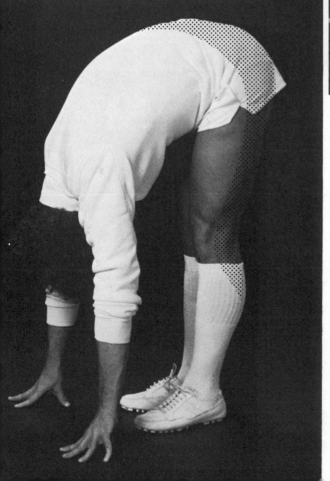

11

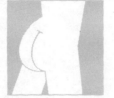

Tushies

─────London Dairy Air─────

Tushies are very important culturally. After all, they are the first thing the doctor slaps when he welcomes you into the world and the last thing you rest on when you say goodbye. In between those two big events you will use your tushy for a lot of sitting, a lot of pairs of blue jeans, and maybe even a bit of wiggling.

You might as well know this right up front: 1984 is going to be the year of the tush. Jiggle is passé. Trim is in. I can tell from watching television. Have you seen that Underalls commercial? Look around you. What do you see? A return to the 1950's. Lots of old pictures of Marilyn Monroe. Voluptuous is returning. So, if your buns aren't shapely enough, you've got only two choices: (1) call Frederick's of Hollywood, I think they make underpants that are padded; or (2) pull out your exercise mat and get to work.

When I worked on *General Hospital*, there was so much interest in buns that we finally sat down during lunch one day and had a buns contest on the disco set. Male cast and crew alike were invited to dance (no one wanted to eat when they saw the competition) while the women judged. Tony Geary came in first place, someone from the lighting department came in second, and I came in third. (The second-place winner went from the lighting booth into an acting job in a matter of weeks. Can you guess who it is? Send me your guess c/o PO Box 5403, Beverly Hills, California, 90210.)

It's unlikely that the current interest in buns will subside. Think of all the names society has already coined for this one part of the anatomy:

tushy
buns
fanny
cheeks
butt
behind
derriere
seat
rump
bottom
backside
bum
ass

If you can think of any others, write them in here:

_____

_____

_____

_____

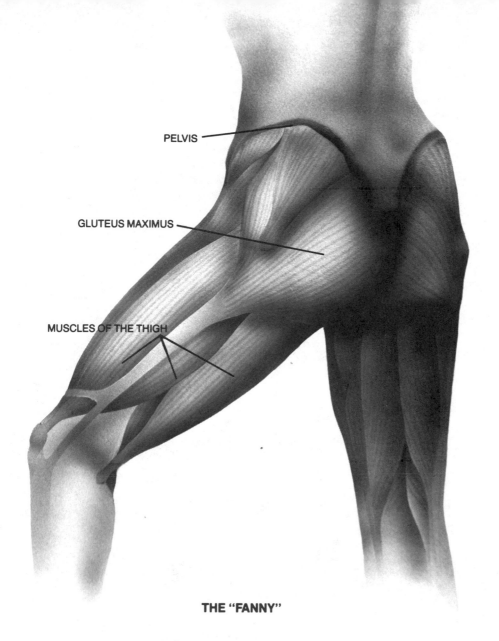

PELVIS

GLUTEUS MAXIMUS

MUSCLES OF THE THIGH

THE "FANNY"

Fanny Dynamics

Most of us sit on our fannies all day long. We don't exercise them, we just put weight on them. Do you realize that a woman who weighs one hundred twenty-five pounds is putting eighty-five pounds of weight on her rear end when she's sitting? No wonder she's worried about spreading acreage. If you sit too much, you'll have bun breakdown. After all, the fanny is composed of muscles. If those muscles get weak, fat deposits run wild and you get wider, thicker, flabbier rear ends.

While structurally the buns are made up of the same muscles that comprise the thighs, we always think of the thighs as the upper part of the leg and the buns as what we sit on.

Your basic buns builders are located right behind your pelvic girdle. The size of your fanny is dependent on:

• the width of your pelvic girdle (women's are automatically wider than men's).
• genes (heredity always counts for something).
• the ratio of fat to muscles.
• weight control during pregnancy.
• exercise and the size of the muscles themselves.

You can trim and tone your backside at the same time that you work on your hips and your thighs.

T1 Minilifts

***Position:** on mat, lying on back, hands at your sides.*

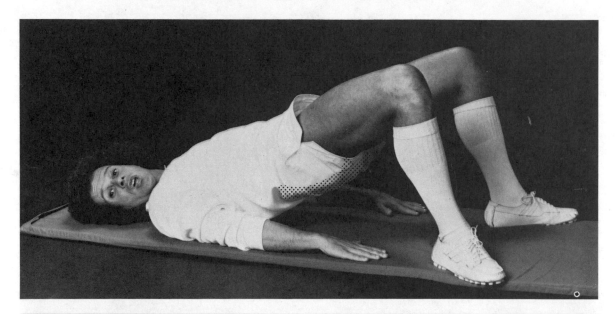

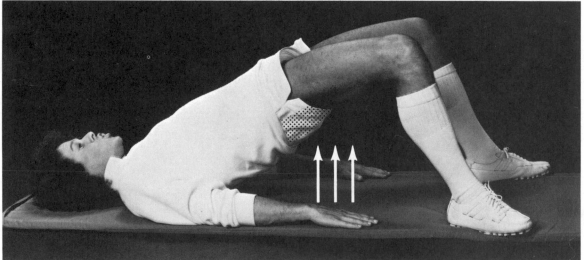

1. With knees bent, slowly lift your back up off the mat.

2. Slowly lower yourself to the mat.

T2 Buttock Tucks

Position: on mat, lying on back, hands at your sides.

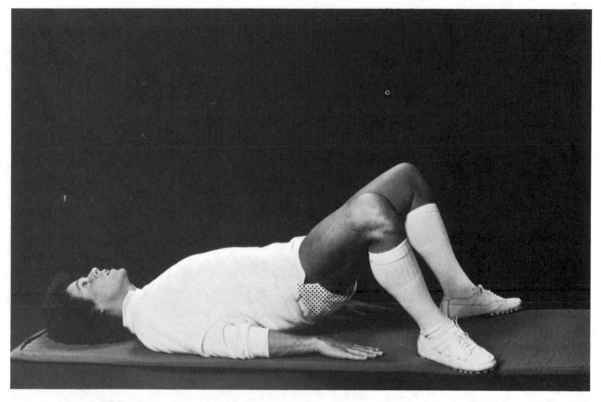

1. **Keep knees bent and feet flat on the floor.**

2. **Keep lower back on the floor.**

3. **Raise your buns up into the air. Tighten those muscles as you lift.**

T3 *Lifts with Knees and Feet Apart*

Position: on mat, lying on back, hands at your sides.

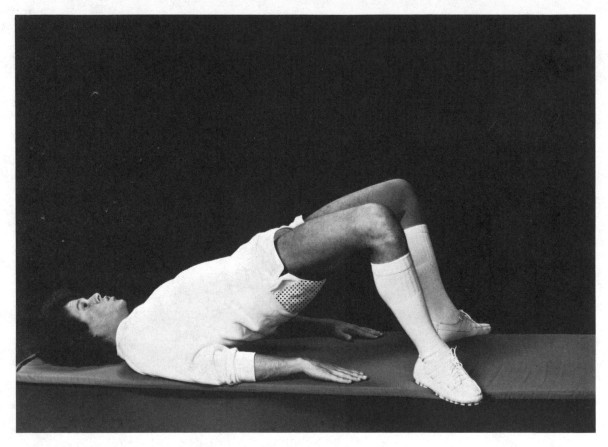

1. Keep knees bent and knees and feet far apart.

2. Turn your feet out.

3. Lift your buns and squeeze those muscles.

T4 Lifts with Knees Together, Feet Apart

Position: on mat, lying on back, hands at your sides.

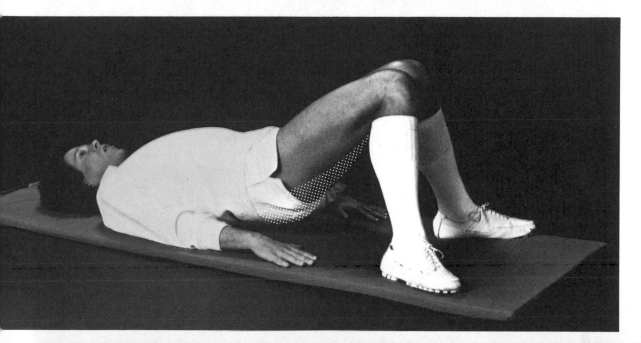

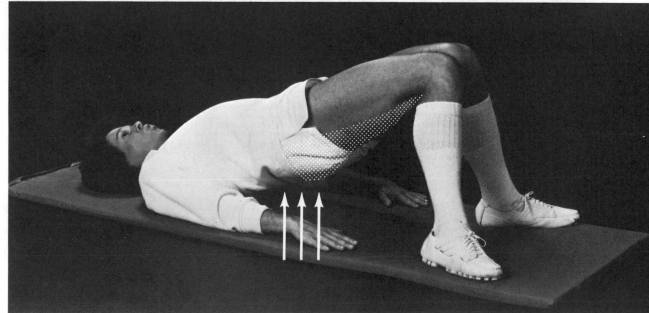

1. **Keep knees bent and together and feet apart.**

2. **Lift your buns and squeeze those muscles.**

T5 *Lifts with Knees and Feet Together*

Position: on mat, lying on back, hands at your sides.

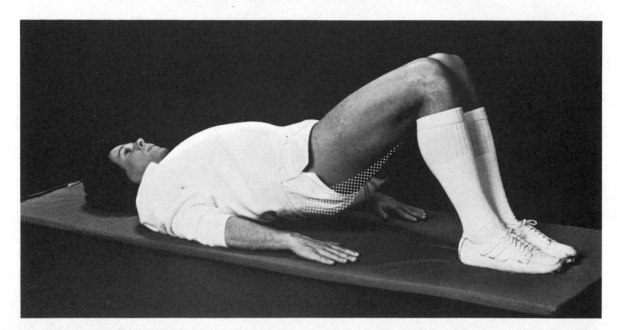

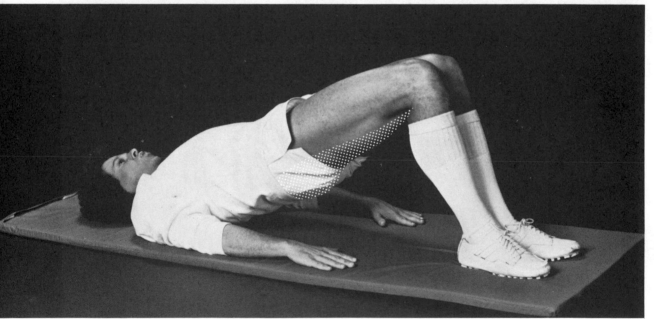

1. **Keep knees and feet together.**

2. **Heels shouldn't be too close to your buns and should be on the floor.**

3. **Lift your buns and squeeze those muscles.**

T6 Hip Swings

Position: on mat, lying on back, hands at your sides.

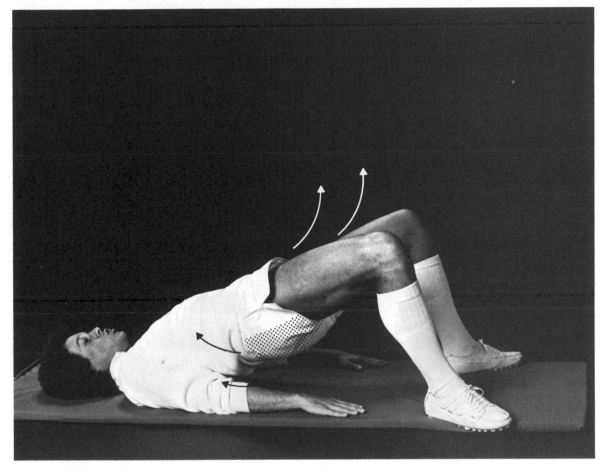

1. **Keep feet and knees apart.**

2. **Shoulders and upper back should be down.**

3. **Lift lower back and buns and swing from side to side gently.**

T7 *Alternating Lifts*

Position: on mat, lying on stomach.

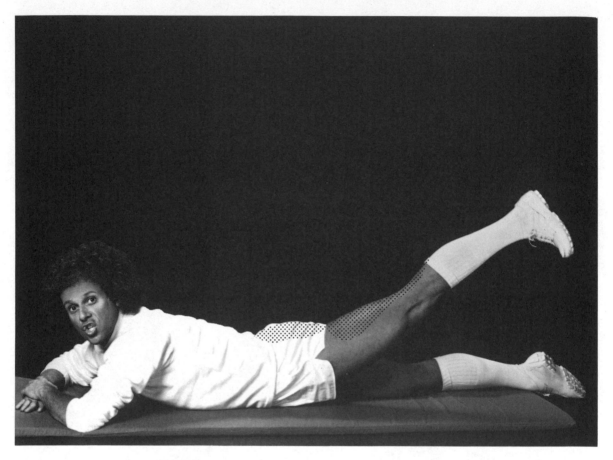

1. Leaning on elbows, lift one leg up at a time.

2. Alternate legs.

T8 Double Alternating Lifts

Position: on mat, lying on stomach.

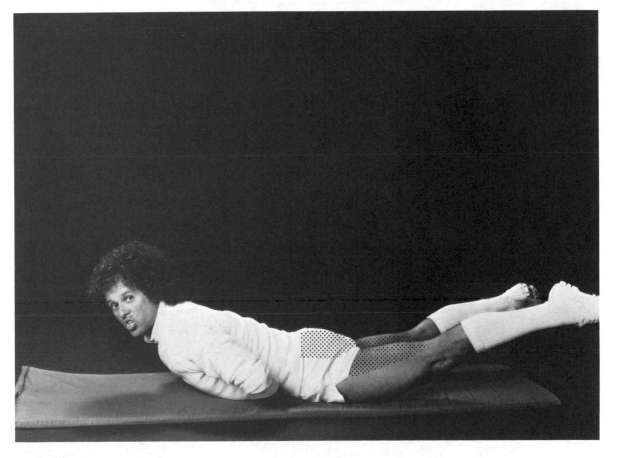

1. **Put your hands under your pelvic bones and lift both legs up at the same time.**

2. **Raise legs so thighs are off the mat.**

3. **Point your toes, lift, release, lift, release, without putting feet to the ground.**

T9 Heel Claps

Position: on mat, lying on stomach.

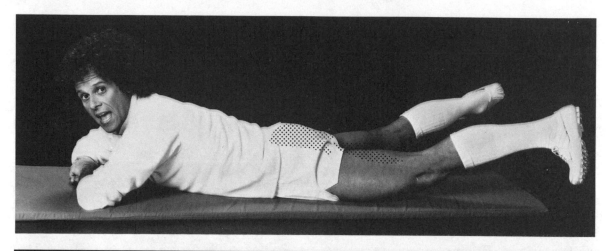

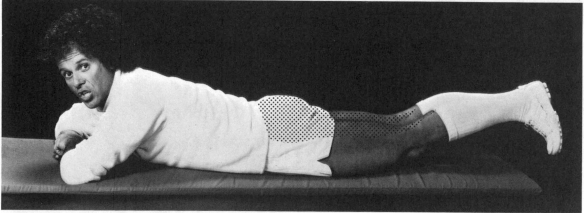

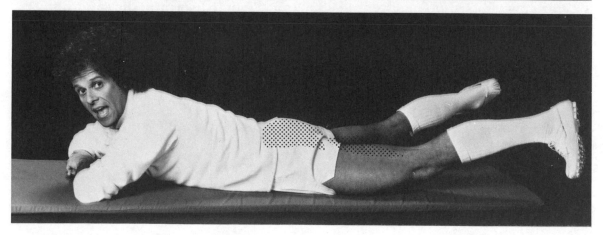

1. Hands can be under pelvic bones as before, or you may rest on your elbows.

2. Lift both legs at the same time, squeezing your heels together. Release heels and squeeze again. (Yes, of course you look like a seal in the circus. So does everyone else who does this one.)

T10 Lifts (Point and Flex)

Position: on mat, lying on stomach.

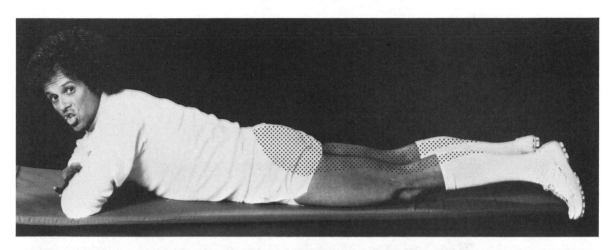

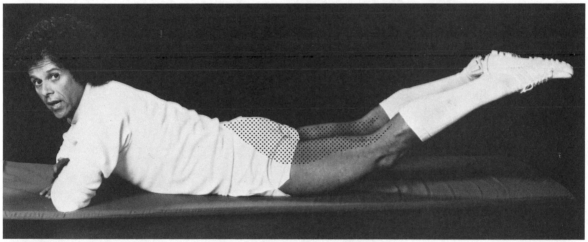

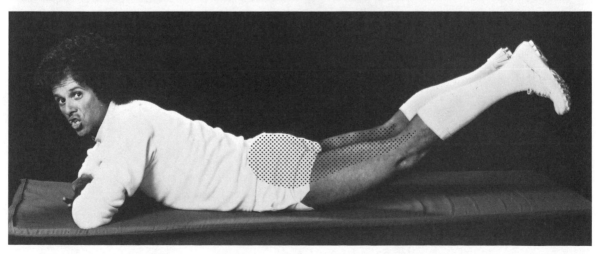

1. Leaning on elbows, lift both legs at same time and point and flex, point and flex.

12

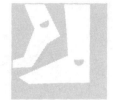

Feet

Put Your Right Foot in and
You Shake It All Around

There are several good things about feet, and one of the best is that there are two of them. I'm just going to discuss the medical aspects of one foot now, but I assure you, everything I say applies to both feet.

This is a foot.

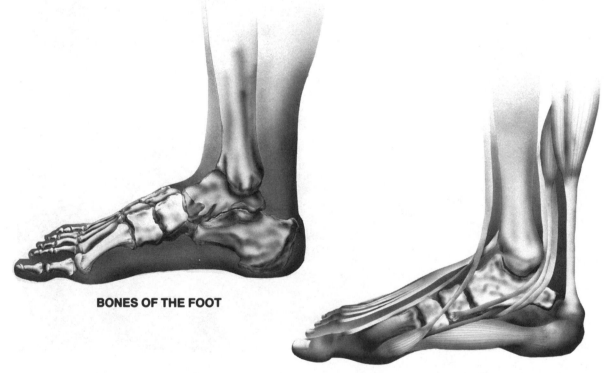

BONES OF THE FOOT

**MUSCLES OF THE FOOT
(AND CALF)**

You'll probably be very interested in some foot facts that you have never considered before:

• The sole of the foot and the palm of the hand have a good bit in common. Both are excellent means of identification as well. (In the state of California a child's birth certificate includes a set of his footprints taken at birth. It looks like a mouse walked across a piece of paper.)

• The bones of the footsie work together to bear the weight of the body, so losing weight is being nice to your feet. If you are extremely heavy and can't lose weight, consider growing another pair of legs.

• Your feet are mainly responsible for your sense of balance.

• There are fourteen phalanges (digital bones) per foot and seven tarsal bones, which make your feet the boniest part of your body.

• The foot is one head in length.

• Most of the muscles for the feet and toes are actually in the calf—only the tendons are in the foot.

• There is a wide discrepancy of toe sizes among people: Some have large big toes, some have longer second toes, some have toes all the same size. This may be heredi-tary, so look at your mother's toes next time you see her.

• The soles or bottoms of your feet are actually formed by fat, which is the best place in your body to be fat!

• During World War I you could not pass the draft physical if you had flat feet, because it was thought harmful for you to march long distances. In World War II men with flat feet were drafted, because in the intervening peacetime years studies proved that flat-footed people were least likely to suffer. But when the guys at the draft board took a look at my flat feet, they put a big 4-F on my report card.

• Feet suffer more circulation problems than any other part of the body.

• Ectomorphs (see page 5; you remember them, don't you?) are lighter on their feet and have a more agile walk than endomorphs. Mesomorphs have the most athletic walk of all three body types.

• Many diseases can first be spotted from the condition of the feet, including diabetes.

• Standing is more tiring than walking.

• The average size of a woman's foot is eight inches and a man's is eleven inches. Isn't that enough to convert you to metric?

Barefoot and Pregnant

While most of the pregnant women I see are wearing high heels or running shoes, the old expression "barefoot and pregnant" has stuck. It's probably because as the pregnancy progresses many women find that their feet swell. Their old shoes feel tight, so they take them off. Hence they are barefoot and pregnant!

Most feet problems—swelling, cramping, varicose veins—disappear after the baby is born and are not serious. But the condition of your feet while you are with child can affect how well you feel, so take notes, please.

1. If your shoes are tight because your feet have swollen, buy two new pairs and alternate them each day.

2. Keep your weight gain to the specifications of your doctor. The more you gain, the more you have to lose later. (The baby won't be born weighing in at fifty pounds!) The strain of extra weight directly affects how your legs and feet feel.

3. Wear low, broad heels that feel comfortable. If you are used to wearing spike heels, the muscles in your legs may have shortened over the years so that lower heels

will hurt you. (This is not uncommon.) Choose shoes that are comfortable.

4. Try maternity-size support panty hose. If they seem to constrict your feet, investigate toeless surgical support hosiery.

5. Foot exercises will help keep up the circulation in your feet. Circulation slows down automatically during pregnancy anyway, and your feet are the farthest from your heart. So don't forget to give them a workout and then elevate them at the end of the day.

6. Never wear any clothing or fashion item that might constrict circulation. Leg warmers should be loose-fitting.

7. Just about the time you can't see your feet, get a pedicure. It'll make you feel glamorous.

On Your Feet

People who sit at a desk all day often complain about *secretarial spread*—a polite term for a broad beam. But people who are on their feet all day—bank tellers, waitresses, mailmen, construction workers—know how important their feet are to their ability to perform their jobs well.

Some people have weak feet and end up with problems only after they undertake foot-stress jobs. Others develop problems on the job. Sometimes there are several small injuries that go unnoticed until one straw breaks the camel's back. And you don't have to be out of the home to suffer from foot injuries. There's a bedroom fracture that doctors are familiar with that occurs when a person gets out of bed in the middle of the night (for a midnight snack?), doesn't turn on a light, and knocks into a piece of furniture or trips and falls, thus injuring the foot.

So whether you're a housewife, a hairdresser, or a meter maid, here are some tips to help protect your feet and keep you more comfortable.

- If you are overweight, lose weight.
- Make sure you have good posture.
- If your feet are exposed to wet, damp, or humid conditions while you are standing all day, install slat boards so your shoes (and feet) rest on the boards rather than on the dampness.
- Move your feet whenever possible, even if you just walk in place.
- If you are standing still, try putting your weight on the outer border of your feet while your toes still point straight ahead.
- Wear shoes that are comfortable and that give good support. Never attempt to break in a pair of shoes. They must feel great when you try them on in the shoe store.
- Take frequent breaks to detense your feet—do exercises, massage your feet, walk (roll) on a rolling pin.
- Don't wear the same shoes every day. Alternate between two pairs, even if the shoes are identical.

FT1 Toe Pulls

Position: on mat, sitting up with straight back.
(I dare you to find this exercise in any other book.)

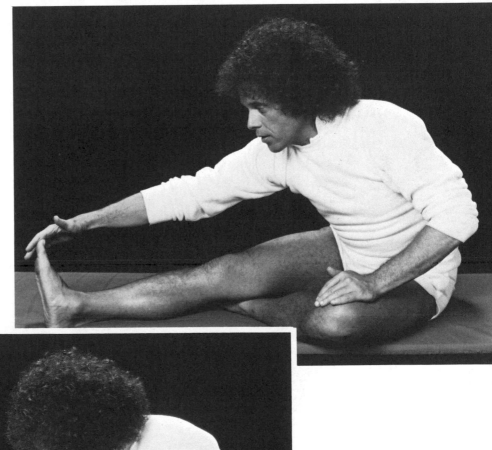

1. **Keep one leg bent, one straight out in front of you.**

2. **Use your hands to curl your toes in toward you.**

3. **Alternate legs.**

FT2 Hammer Toes

Position: standing, one leg straight, one leg bent.

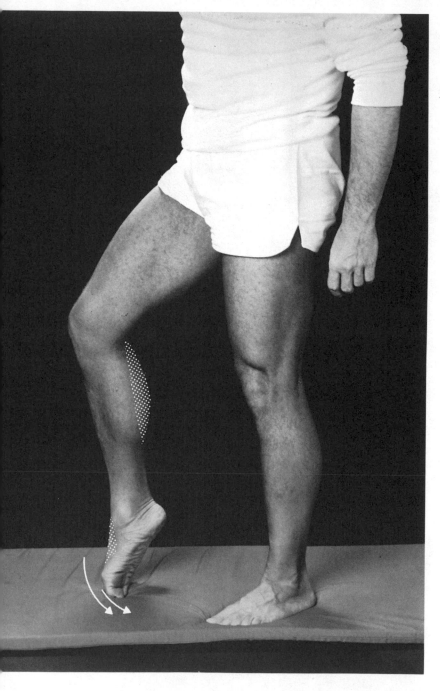

1. Bend right knee and push toes into mat, curling them under to the toe knuckles, or whatever they call those joints.

2. Alternate legs.

FT3 Ankle Rotations

Position: on mat, sitting up, legs bent.

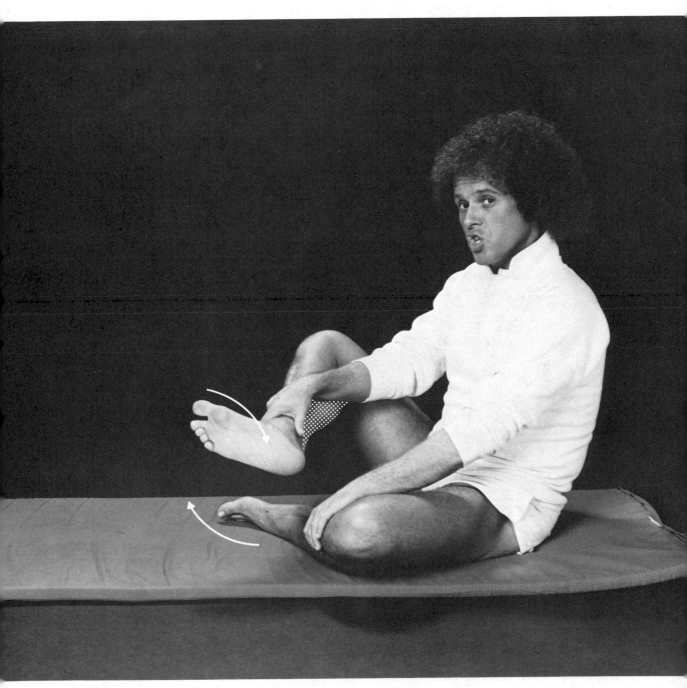

1. Using your arms to support yourself, raise legs, bend your knees, and circle your ankles around at the joints (one at a time, please).

2. Reverse rotation.

FT4 Toe Fans *(This is not what tofu is. I said Toe Fans—Toe Fans.)*

Position: on mat, sitting up. (Do not do this wearing panty hose or tights with toes.)

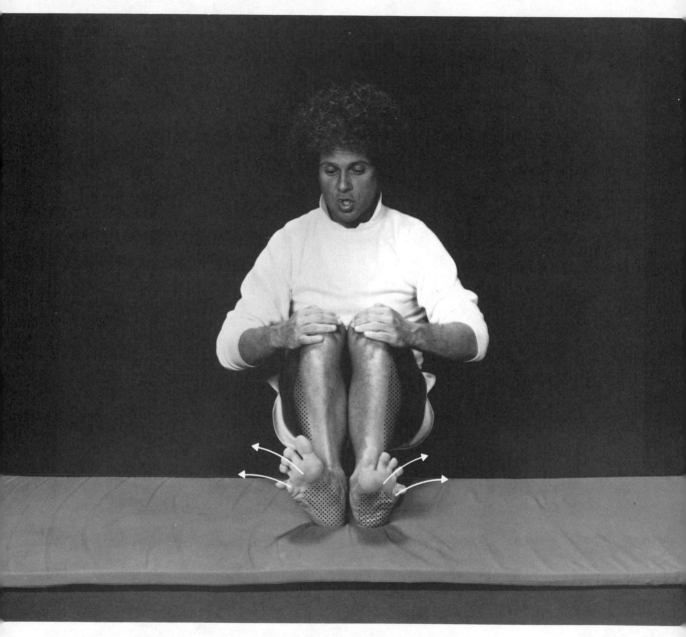

1. Legs are straight out in front of you. (Okay, bend if you want.)

2. Spread your toes as wide open as you can.

3. Hold the fans and release.

FT5 Feet Rows

Position: on mat, sitting up.

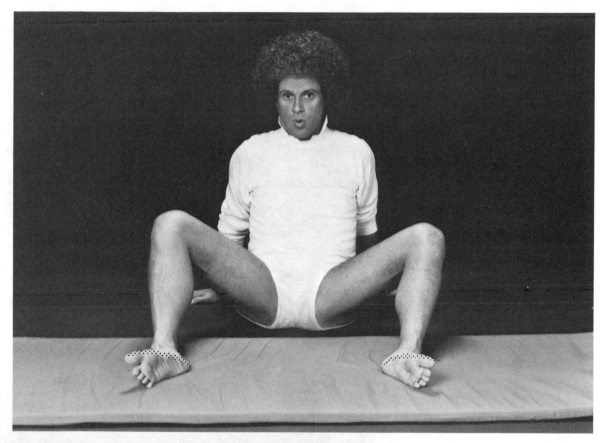

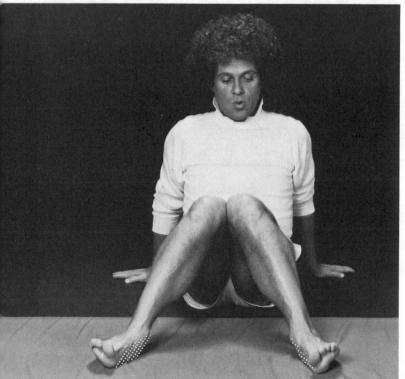

1. Spread legs, bend knees, and place feet down on the mat.

2. Roll your feet from side to side as you open and close your legs while you sing "Row, Row, Row Your Boat."

FT6 Sock Crawlers

Position: standing.

1. Take a clean sock and, using your toes, squeeze it up.

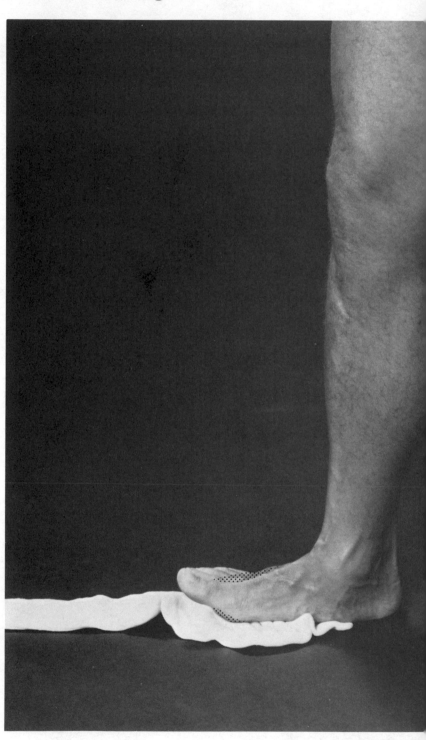

FT7 Double Sock Crawlers

Position: standing.

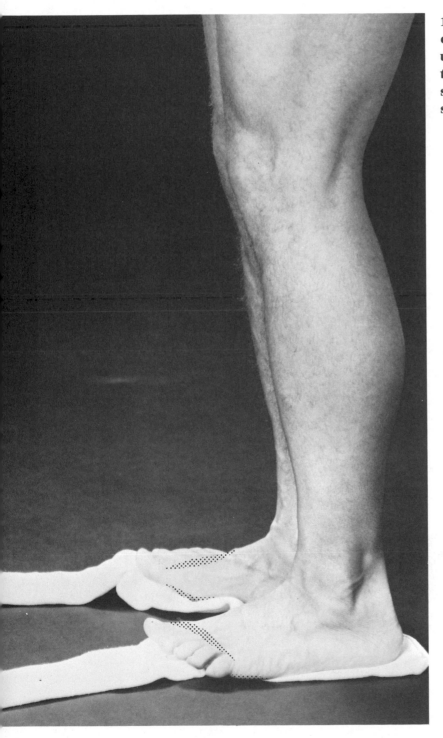

1. Take two clean socks—one for each foot—and, using your toes, squeeze them up with both feet at same time. (Have you ever seen such talent?)

FT8 Arch Rolls

Position: standing.

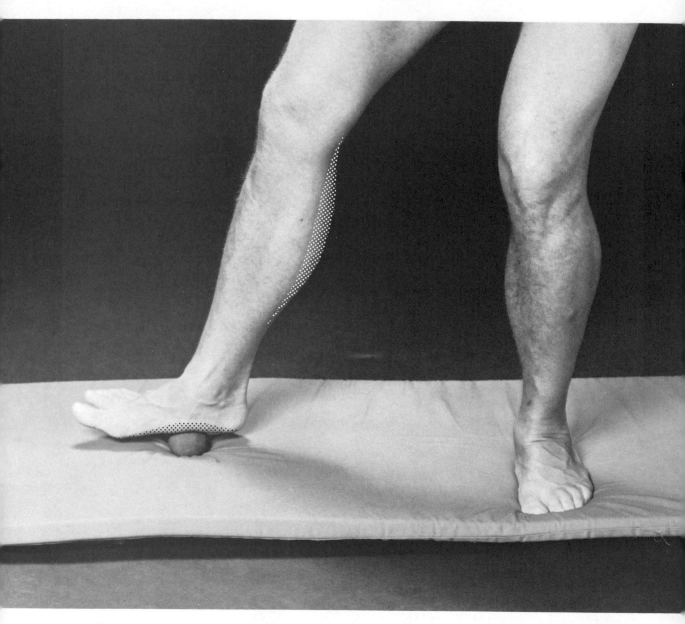

1. Roll a small ball under your foot, using the arch to roll the ball. You can do this with an imaginary ball.

2. Alternate feet.

FT9 Foot Massage

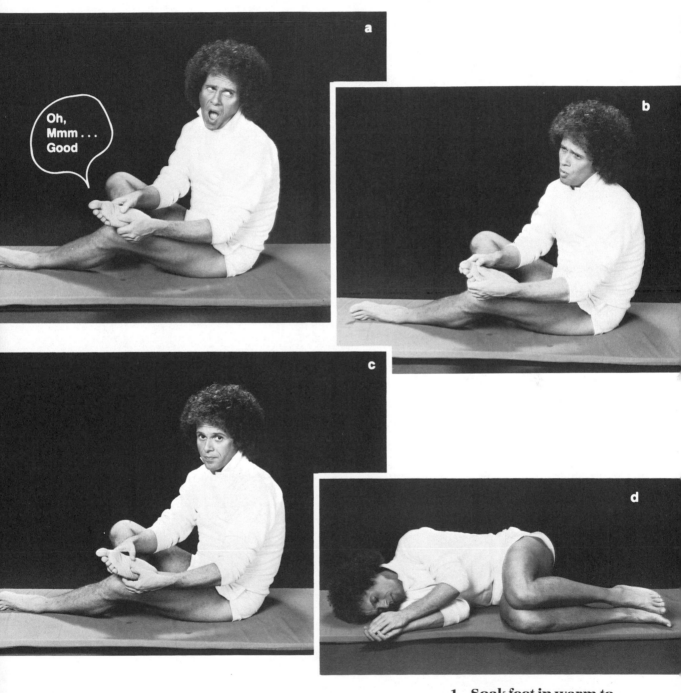

1. **Soak feet in warm to hot water.**

2. **Use baby oil as you massage your feet gently with your hands.**

Special Programs

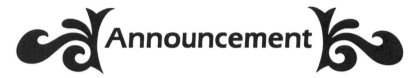# Announcement

Some exercise gurus will tell you to do ten of these and six of these and twenty-seven of those until you're ready to build up by fours. Well, sorry, folks, but I can't go through life counting things. If you are a beginner, you begin at the beginning. Do a little. Do what you can. Then build up slowly. If it starts to hurt, quit for now. Do a little more each day. The goal is never to do less than what you did the day before. If you copped out and missed a day or two, of course, go back. The body stays in shape for only three days, remember. But in some of the programs you will find the number of suggested repetitions. Try to work up to that number and make sure your body feels good about doing that many before you go on to the next step.

The first three programs in this section are progressive, so when one gets easy for you, go on to another. Do what you can, and always do more than the time before.

And remember to begin and end each program with some deep breathing.

Beginner Program

If you are not exercising three to four hours a week (and I don't mean playing sports or going to the grocery store), you are a BEGINNER. This is not bad news. This is nothing to be upset about. Almost everyone reading this book is a BEGINNER.

Sure, you can do some arm circles and a couple of sit-ups. But you do not have the strength or the flexibility to do an hour's worth of exercise properly and without being very, very sore. Don't feel bad. It's better to be a great BEGINNER than a struggling INTERMEDIATE. Start small and build up. Remember when you were at summer camp and that the first day you were afraid to go in the pool, yet by the time your parents came you won the Minnewonka Swim? Show me that same old spirit.

Stay in the BEGINNER program at least four weeks. If you have a lot of weight to lose, you may stay longer.

F10 4 times   **F11** 4 times   **F12** 8 times   **SH1** 8 times

SH2 8 times   **W5** 16 times   **ST4** 8 times   **W3** 8 times

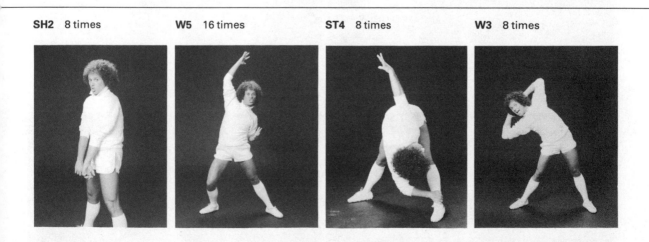

W7 8 times

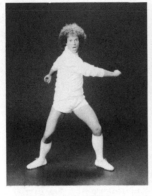

W8 8 times

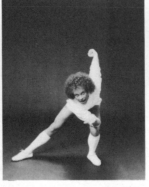

B5 8 times

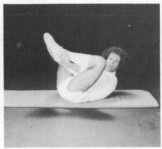

H1*

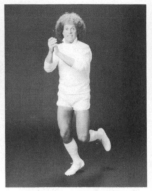

H2*

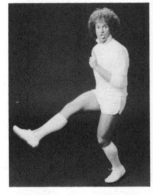

H3*

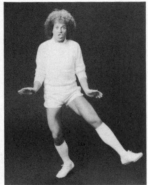

H4*

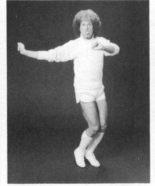

H5*

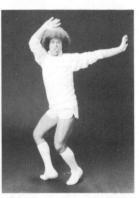

H6*

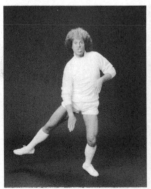

H7*

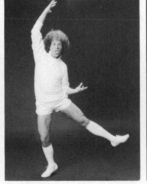

H1* Cool Down

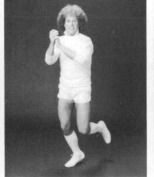

A2 8 times
forward and back

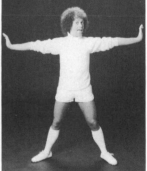

*These exercises combined should take five minutes.

A14 8 times

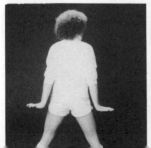

A10 8 times

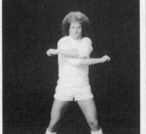

A13 8 times

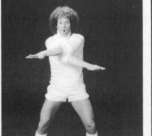

A12 8 times

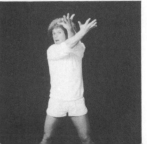

A18 8 times

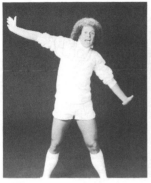

C5 8 times

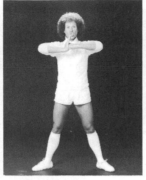

HT1 4 times

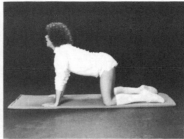

HT2 8 times

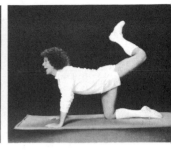

HT5 8 times

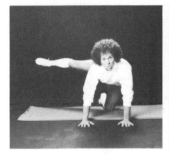

HT7 8 times

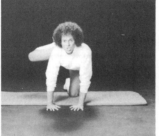

HT12 8 times

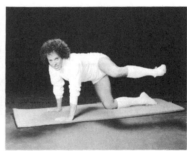

W3 8 times
Hold for Stretch

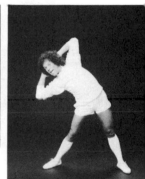

ST9 8 times

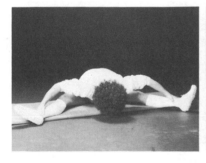

ST11 8 times

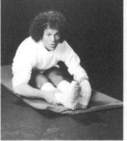

S2 8 times

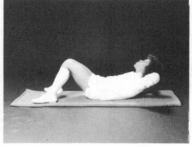

S17 8 times

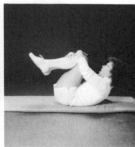

S2 8 times

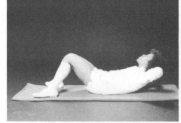

S7 8 times

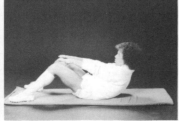

S17 8 times

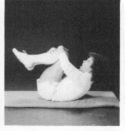

S19 8 times

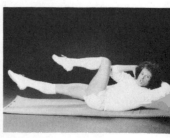

S17 8 times

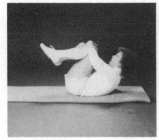

S19 8 times

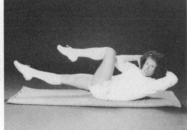

W3 8 times

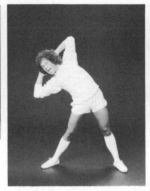

T2 16 times

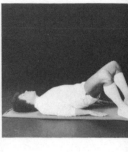

T3 16 times

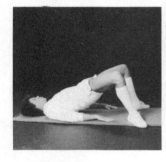

L1 8 times

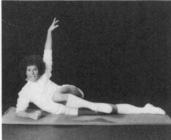

L3 16 times

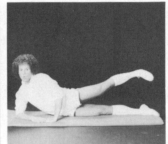

L4 8 times
forward and back

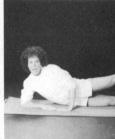

T10 8 times

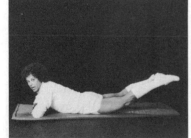

FT1 8 times

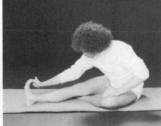

FT2 8 times

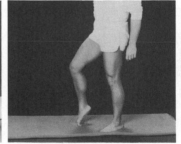

FT9

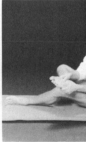

Intermediate Program

Congratulations! You're a little bit stronger than you were a few weeks ago, aren't you? See, you did it! Your stamina is better, you've got more energy, your mobility is better, and you're losing weight. The first thirty days are the hardest, that's true, but you're past that now. This program is a little more difficult, so don't get frustrated. I know you can do it. After all, most people don't even make it past BEGINNER. You'll probably be in this program for about eight weeks, depending on the results you're seeing and what the goals are for your better body. Good for you!

F14 8 times   **F15** 8 times   **F13** 8 times and reverse   **F1** 8 times

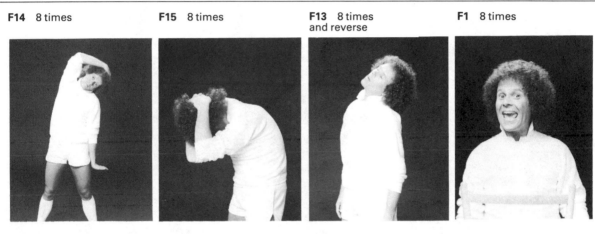

F3 8 times   **F2** 8 times   **F4** 8 times   **SH3** 8 times and reverse

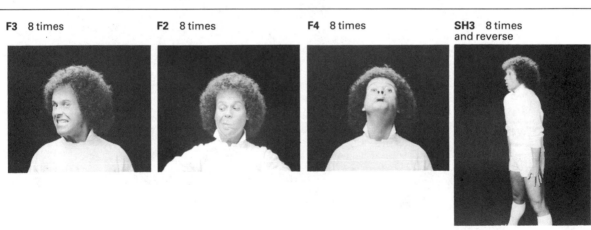

SH6 8 counts

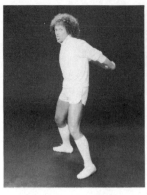

ST5 8 times

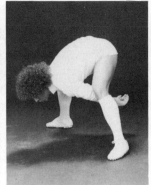

ST4 8 times

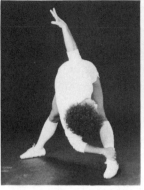

W9 8 times

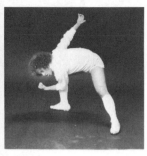

W8 8 times

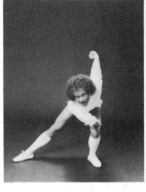

W13 32 times

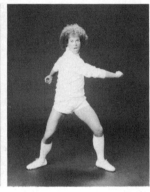

W11 16 times

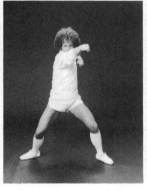

W12 16 times

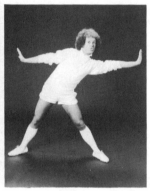

W10 16 times

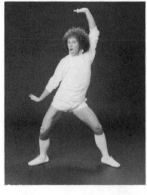

W7 16 times

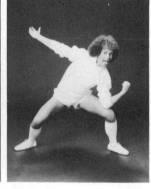

ST11 8 times

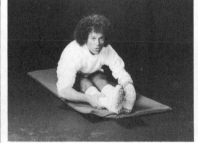

L18 16 times

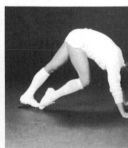

L23 8 times

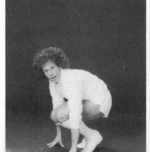

H1*

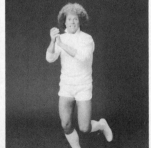

H4*

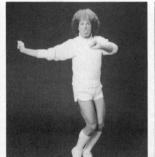

H5*

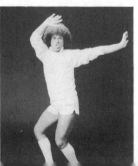

H8*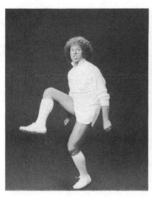

H9*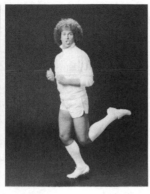

H6*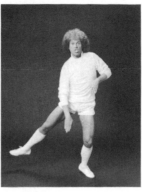

H7*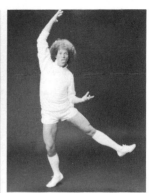

H10*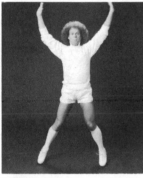

H1* Cool Down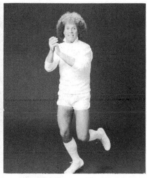

A2 16 times
forward and back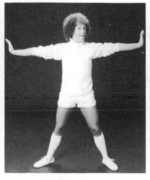

A5 16 times
forward and back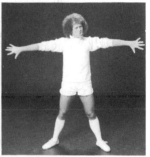

*These exercises combined should take five minutes.

A4 32 times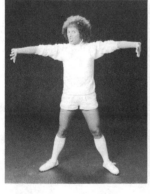

A14 32 times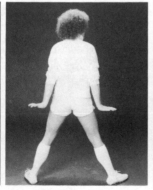

A18 16 times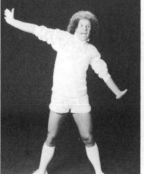

A19 16 times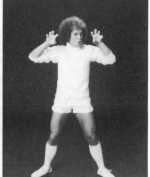

C6 16 times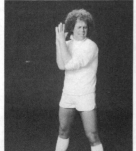

HT1 4 times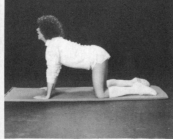

HT2 8 times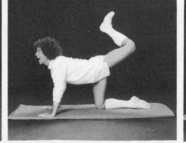

HT3 16 times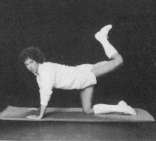

HT4 16 times

HT5 16 times

HT9 16 times

HT10 32 times

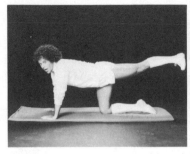
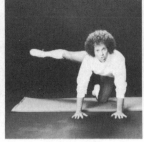
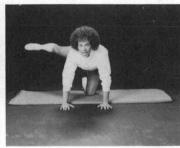
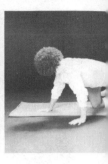

HT1 4 times

C8 16 times

ST14 8 times

ST17 8 times

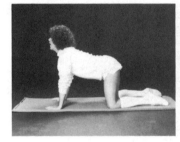
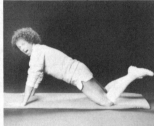
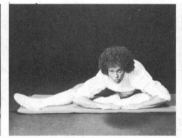
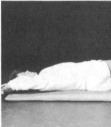

ST9 8 times

ST11 8 times

S1 16 times

S2 16 times

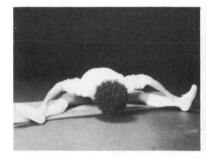
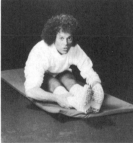
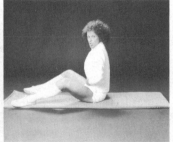
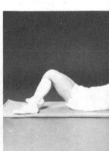

S7 16 times

S17 8 times

S20 16 times

S21 16 times

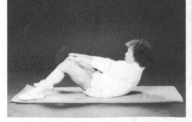
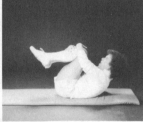
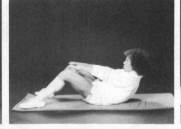
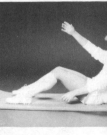

S17 8 times

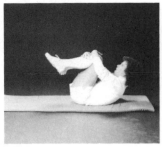

S18 16 times

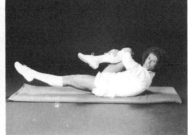

S17 8 counts hold

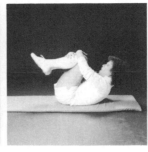

W3 16 times

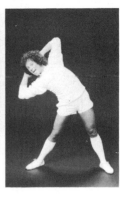

T1 32 times

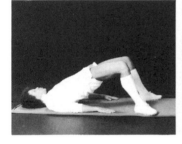

T3 32 times

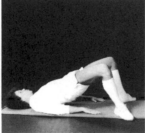

T4 16 times

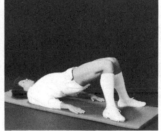

L13 32 times

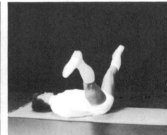

L1 16 times

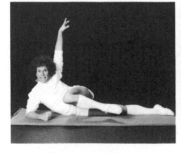

L3 32 times

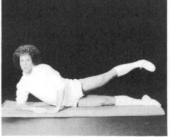

L16 16 times

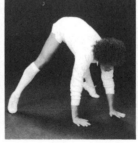

L17 16 times

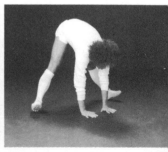

L5 16 times

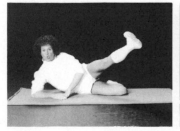

L8 16 times

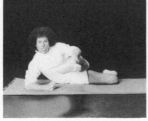

S3 32 times

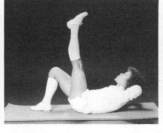

S4 16 times

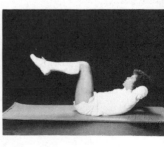

ST1 8 times

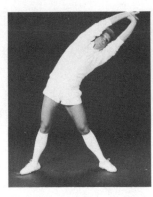

ST9 8 times

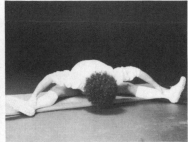

ST12 8 times

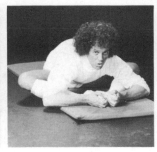

FT1 8 times

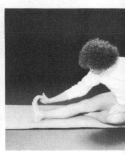

FT8 8 times

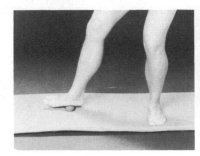

FT9

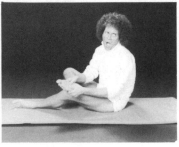

Advanced Program and Maintenance

ADVANCED doesn't mean that you're finished! Oh, no, it just means you've come a long way, baby. Now your body really knows how to work. You don't get sore or tired doing the easy stuff, do you? You've pretty much got your body looking like you want it to, and your heart is pumping a lot better than before. If you've already met all your goals, this is a good maintenance plan for you. If you want to keep going, work with this plan for a few months and then combine it with an aerobics program.

F13 8 times   **F16** 8 times   **F17** 8 times   **F14** 8 times

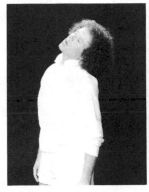 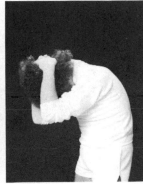 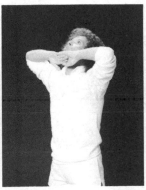 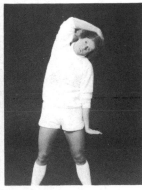

F3 16 times   **F2** 16 times   **F4** 16 times   **F6** 16 times

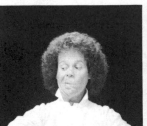 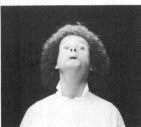 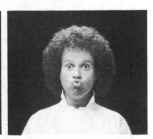

F9   16 times

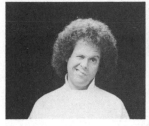

SH3   16 times

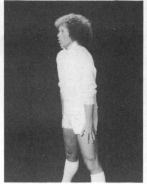

SH5   8 times

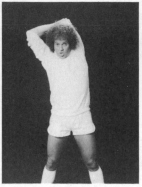

SH7   16 times

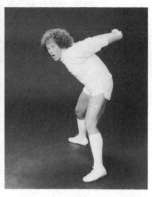

L16   32 times

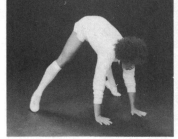

L17   8 times

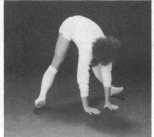

L19   32 times

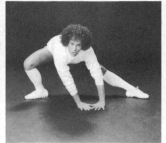

L20   16 times

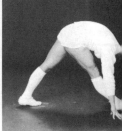

L21   16 times

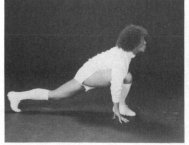

L22   16 times

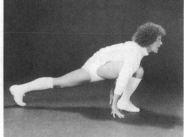

W9   32 times

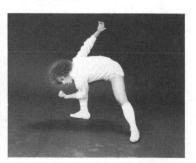

W8   32 times

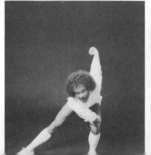

W7   64 times

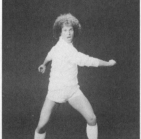

W1   32 times

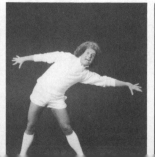

W2   32 times

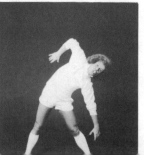

W6 16 times

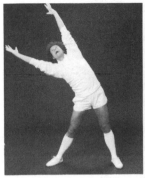

W3 16 times

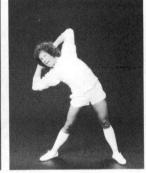

W13 32 times

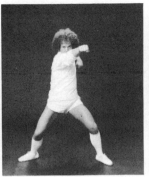

W14 32 times

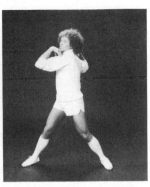

W10 32 times

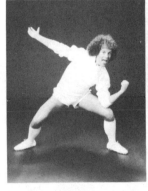

B5 16 times

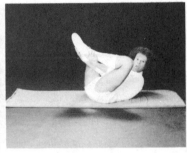

H1*

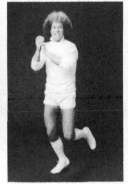

H8*

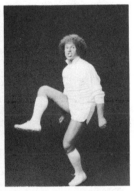

*These exercises combined should take twenty-two minutes.

H4*

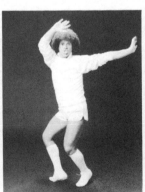

H5*

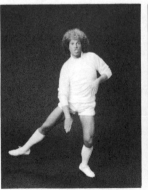

H6*

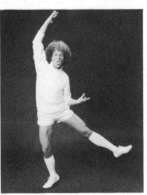

H7*

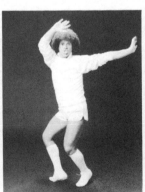

H10*

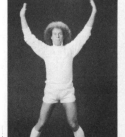

H11*

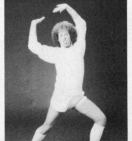

H12*

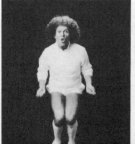

H13*

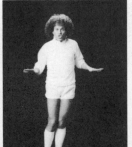

H1* Cool Down

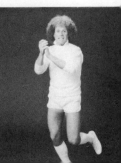

A2 32 times
forward and back

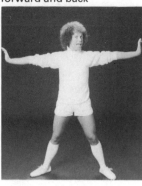

A5 32 times
forward and back

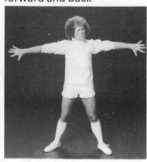

A4 32 times

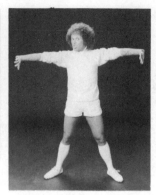

A17 32 times

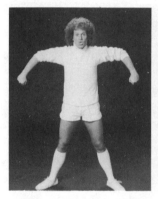

A6 16 times

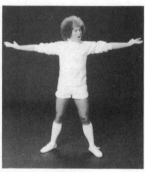

A7 16 times

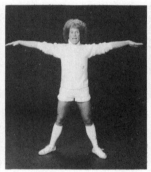

A8 16 times

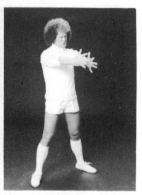

A9 16 times

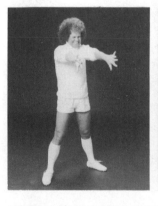

A16 32 times

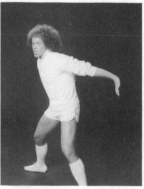

A15 32 times

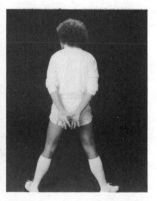

A18 16 times

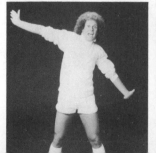

A20 16 times

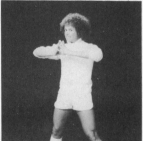

A21 16 times

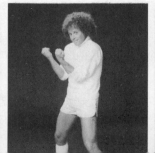

C4 16 times

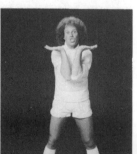

L1   32 times

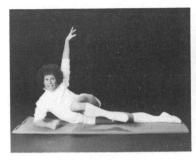

L5   32 times

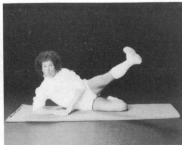

L6   32 times
forward and back

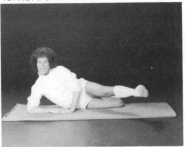

L7   16 times

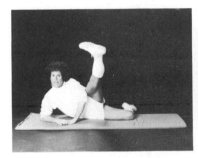

L8   8 times

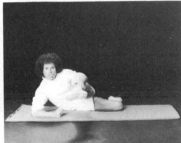

C8   16 times

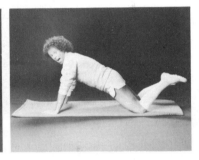

HT3   16 times

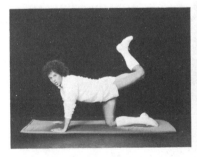

HT4   16 times

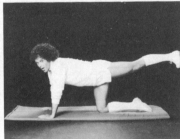

HT5   16 times

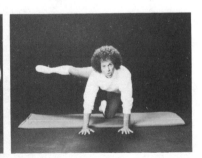

HT12   32 times
forward and back

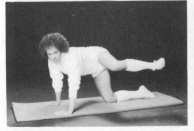

HT7   16 times

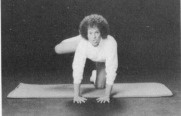

HT8   16
counts hold

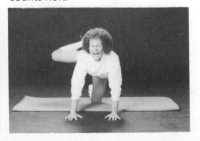

HT10   32 times

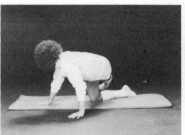

HT11   32 times

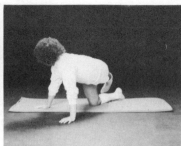

HT1   4 times

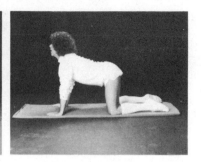

HT14   16 times

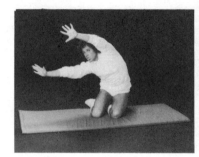

S4   16 times

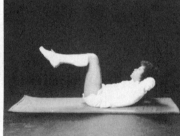

B6   8 counts hold

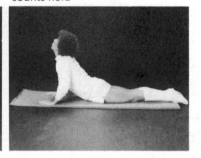

B8   8 counts hold

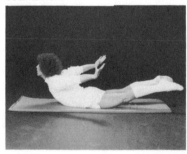

C7   16 times

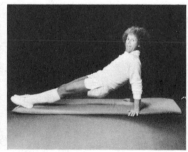

C1   20 times

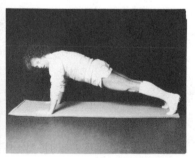

C9   20 times

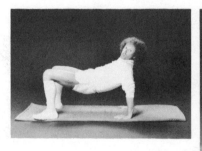

ST3   8 times

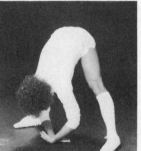

ST4   8 times

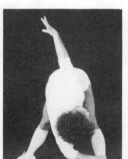

ST10   16 times

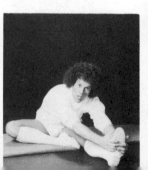

S14 16 times

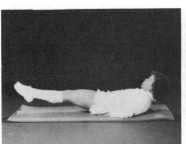

ST10 16 times

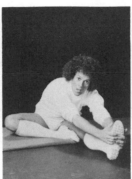

ST9 16 times

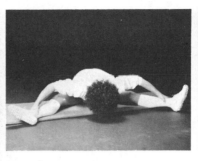

S5 32 times

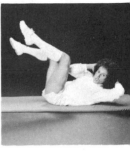

S3 32 times

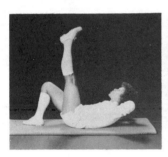

S9 32 times

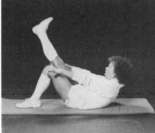

S7 8 times

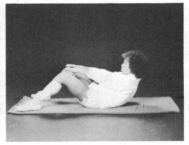

S17 8 times

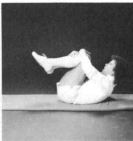

S20 20 times

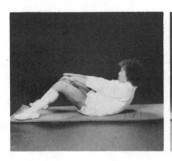

S22 32 times

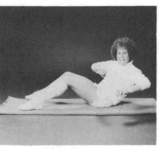

S17 8 times

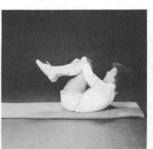

S19 32 times

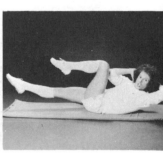

S15 32 times

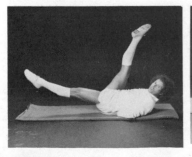

S17 8 times

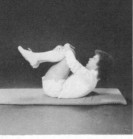

S5 32 times

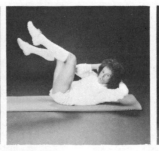

S11 32 times

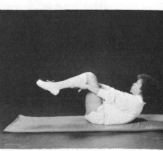

S17 8 times

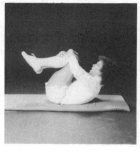

W3 16 times

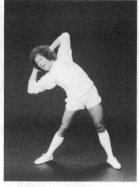

T1 64 times

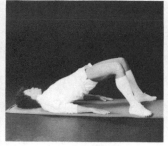

T3 64 times

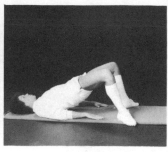

T4 32 times

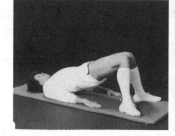

T5 16 times

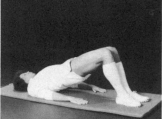

B5 16 times

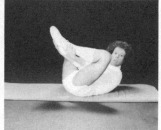

B2 16 times

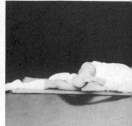

B3 16 times

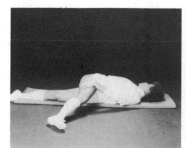

FT1 16 times

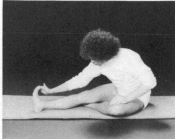

FT6 16 times

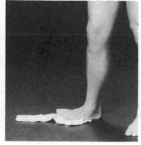

FT9

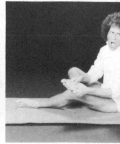

OVERWEIGHTER PROGRAM

If you are fifty pounds or more overweight, you should be in a special exercise class to help you take off weight and get in shape. When you graduate, you will move into the BEGINNER program.

You know, ten years ago a doctor would tell an overweight person not to exercise but to go on a strict food plan and take weight off first. Now doctors' ideas are more modern. I've had OVERWEIGHTER classes for nine years and have found them extremely helpful in motivating a person to lose weight while getting in better physical condition.

The thing for an OVERWEIGHTER to remember above all else is to be patient with your body. You can't move as fast as someone who is lighter, you shouldn't jump around and land on your feet until you've taken off some weight, and you can't get into some of the positions other people can get into until you lose weight. But exercise will help you to reduce. So take your time, concentrate on your food plan and a steady dose of exercise (if you let up for as long as three days, you'll have to start all over again—the body loses tone that quickly), and you will be a winner   and a loser, too! Make sure you exercise in one-hour sessions. It takes thirty minutes to start burning off fat. .

F1 8 times   **F2** 8 times   **F3** 8 times   **F4** 8 times

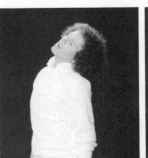 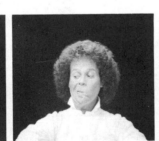 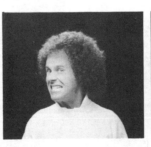 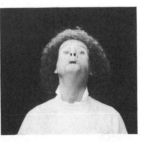

F13 4 times   **SH3** 4 times   **W3** 8 times   **W5** 16 times

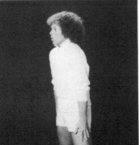 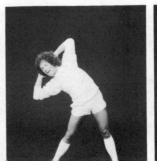 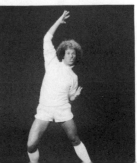

W7 16 times

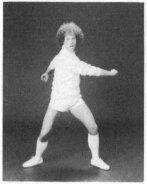

W1 8 times

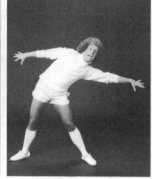

W2 8 times

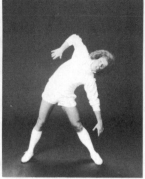

W3 8 times

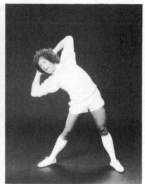

W10 8 times

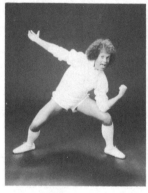

W8 8 times

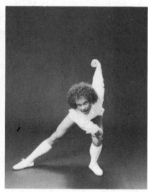

W9 8 times

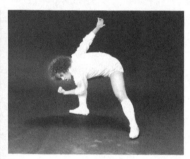

ST4 8 counts

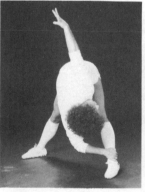

ST5 8 times

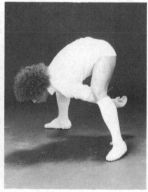

L19 2 counts each side 4 times

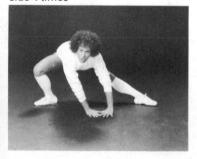

L16 16 times

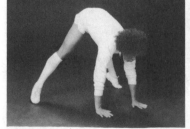

B5 8 times

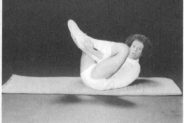

H1*

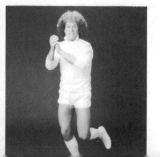

H6*   16 times

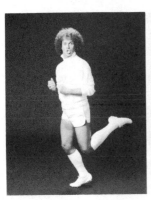

H7*   16 times

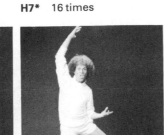

H5*   32 times

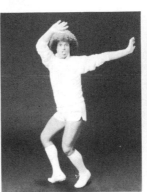

H8*   8 times

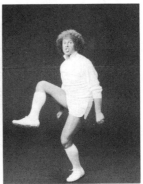

H9*   8 times

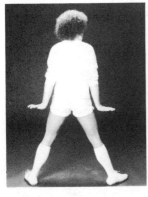

H1*   Cool Down

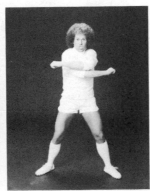

A2   8 times
forward and back

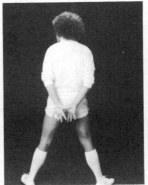

A5   8 times
forward and back

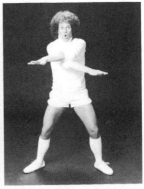

*These exercises combined should take five minutes.

A14   16 times

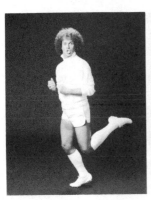

A10   8 times

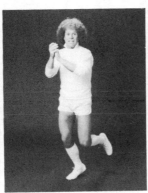

A15   8 times

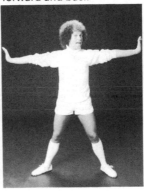

A13   16 times

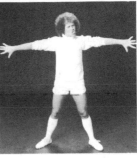

A18   8 times

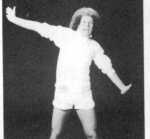

C5   8 times

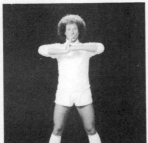

W3   8 times

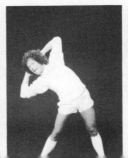

ST9   8 times

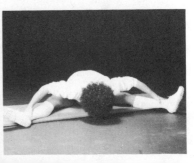

ST11   8 times

HT17   16 times

HT18   8 times

HT19   8 times

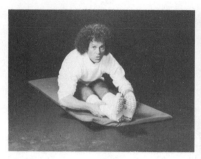
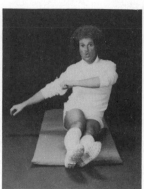
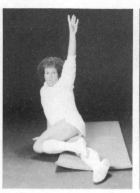
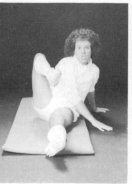

HT1   4 times

HT2   8 times

HT3   16 times

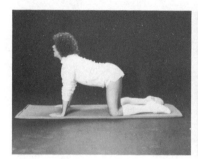
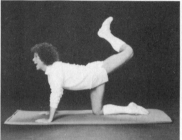
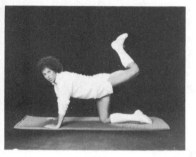

HT7   8 times

HT8   8 times

HT1   4 times

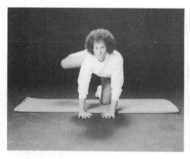
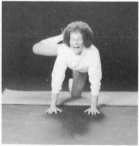
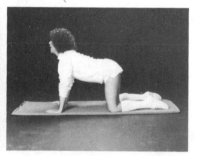

S1   4 times

S2   8 times

S17   8 times

S2   16 times

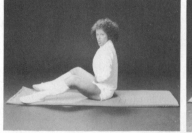
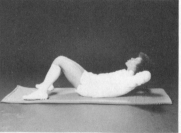
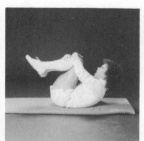
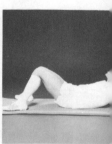

S7 16 times

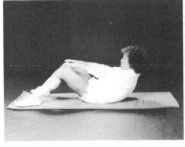

S17 8 times

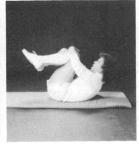

S18 8 times

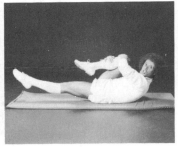

S17 8 times

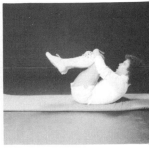

S18 8 times

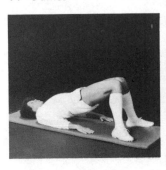

S17 8 times

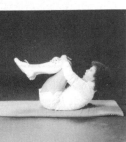

T1 16 times

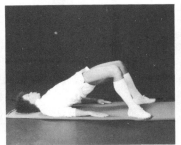

T3 8 times

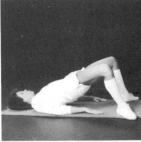

T4 8 times

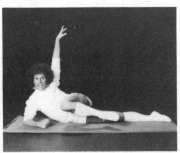

L1 8 times

L3 8 times

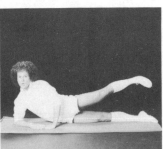

L6 8 times

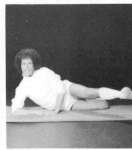

L4 8 times

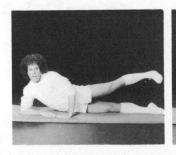

L6 16 times

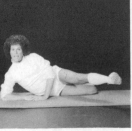

L9 16 times

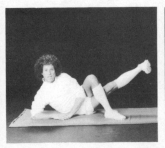

FT1 8 times

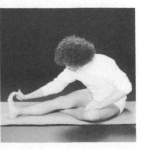

COUPLES PROGRAM

Here's what happens. Mr. and Mrs. Lovely get married and live happily ever after. Except after having three children, Mrs. Lovely finds that she has gained over thirty pounds that she just can't shake. Mr. Lovely has been gaining, too—it's from sitting at a desk all day, he says. Mrs. Lovely goes to class and loses thirty, forty, or fifty pounds and tones and tightens her body. She looks great. What happens? Mr. Lovely freaks out. There is tension in their marriage, and a great thing like weight loss suddenly becomes a terrible thing like treason.

That's why I like the COUPLES program. If you are both overweight, you can lose weight and shape up together. If only one person has a weight problem, you can't tell me that the other person still doesn't need to exercise. Everyone needs to exercise! Going to class makes exercise part of the marriage commitment and part of the partnership. It helps the support system and actually improves the marriage. Why don't you try it and see for yourself?

CO1 Aerobic Twist

Position: standing, facing each other.

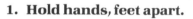

1. **Hold hands, feet apart.**

2. **Jump from side to side (each jump to the opposite side, like doing the hora), keeping knees bent.**

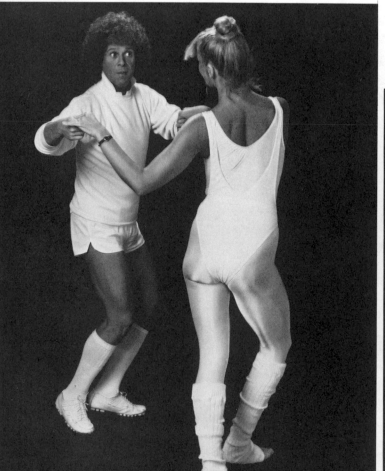

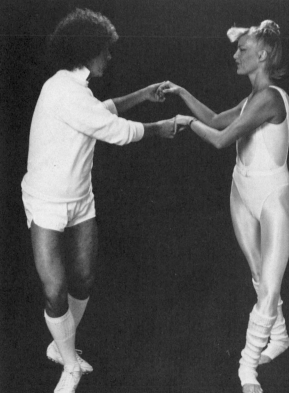

CO2 *Kick Out*

Position: *standing, facing each other.*

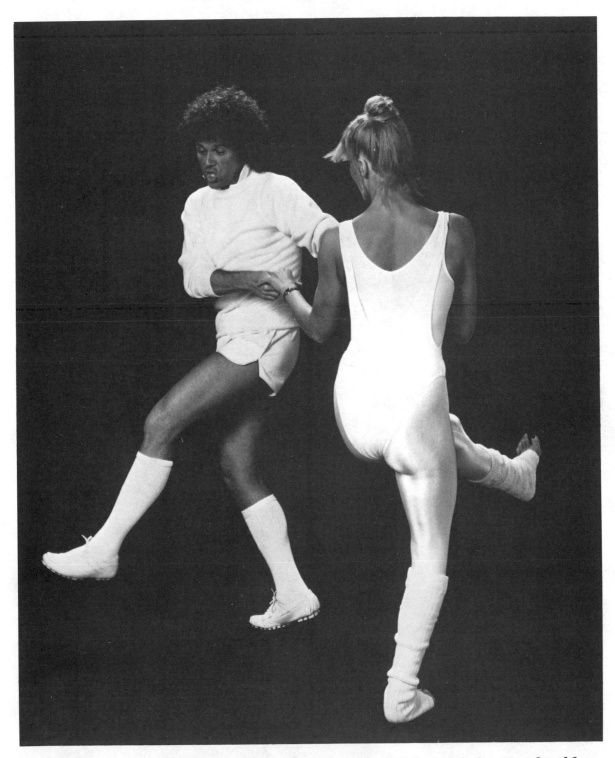

1. Hold hands and twist out to opposite sides, kicking while you twist. You should hop, kick, hop, kick, while still holding hands.

CO3 Arms Out

Position: standing, facing each other.

1. Hold arms out to the sides, placing one hand on top of the other.

2. Push up, then down, alternating hand positions.

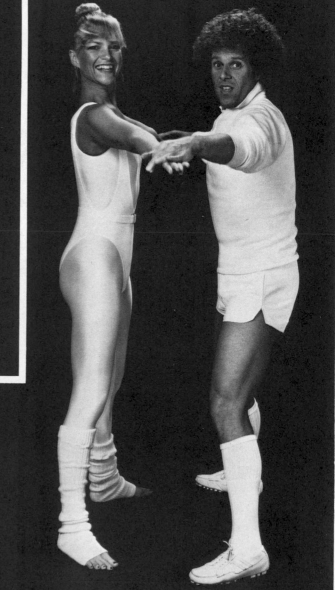

CO4 Push In

Position: standing, facing each other.

1. Hold hands together, straight out in front of you.

2. Push in, then out, alternating hand positions.

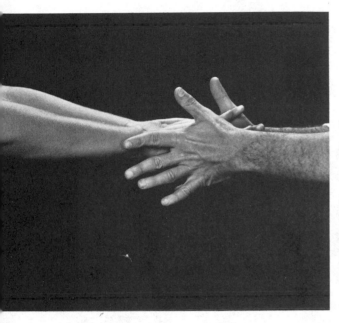

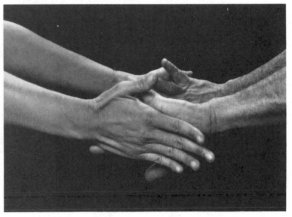

CO5 Bent Elbow Pushes In and Out

Position: standing, facing each other.

1. Bend elbows with hands together.

2. Push in, then out, alternating hand positions.

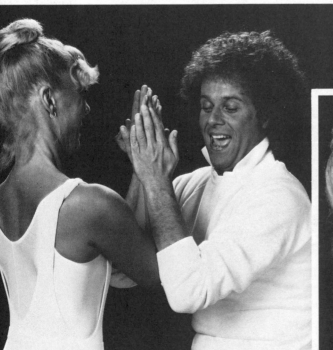

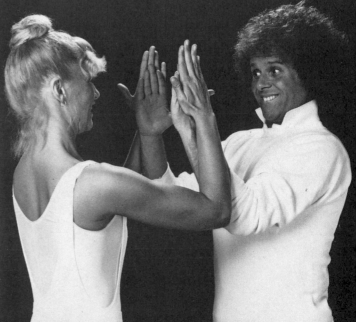

CO6 Couples Straddle Stretch

Position: sitting up on mat, facing each other.

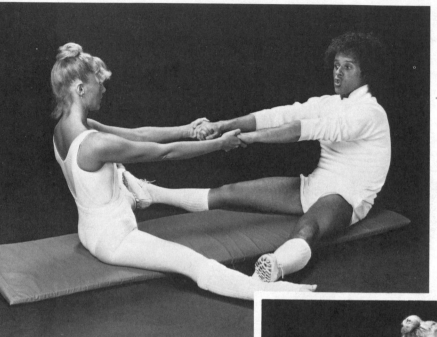

1. Place legs in straddle position, feet touching.

2. Hold hands, then push and pull each other forward and backward.

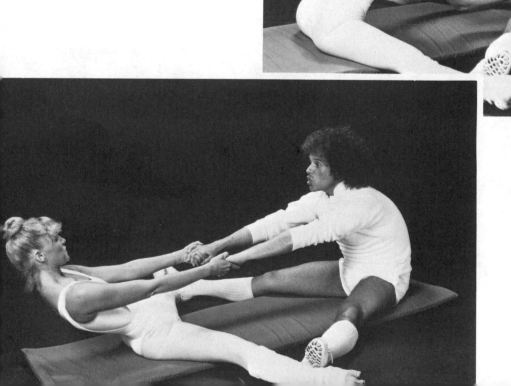

CO7 Buttocks Lifts

Position: lying on mat, one partner's legs between the other's.

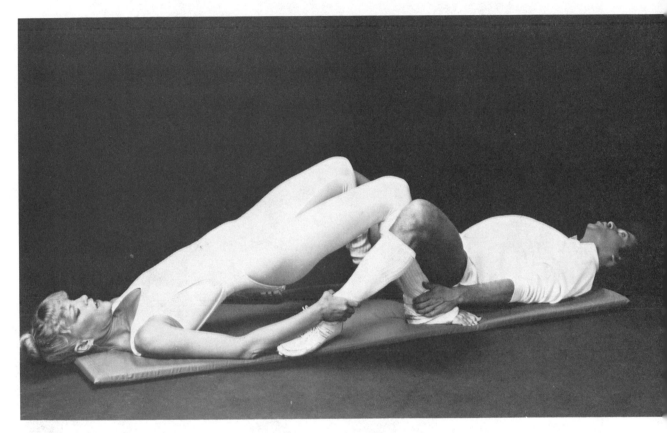

1. Hold each other's ankles while taking turns doing buttocks lifts.

CO8 Couples Forward Back

Position: sitting on mat, back to back.

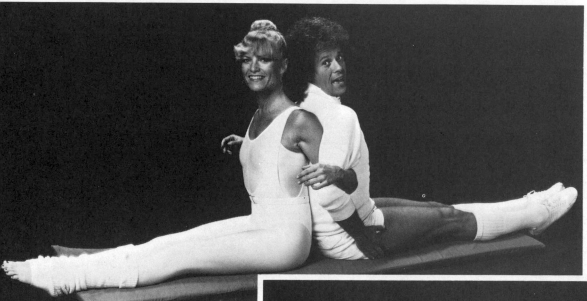

1. **Link arms, then rock forward and backward.**

2. **Keep your necks up and your legs out straight.**

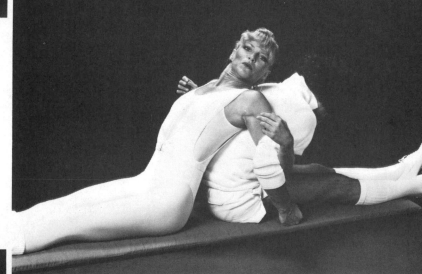

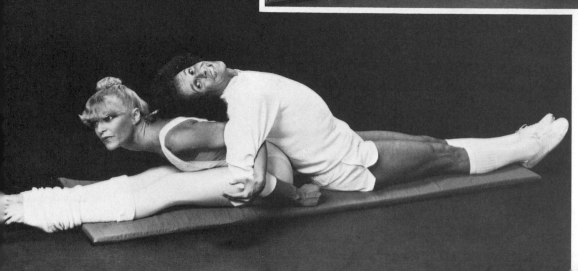

CO9 Side Leg Lifts

Position: lying on sides on mat, facing each other.

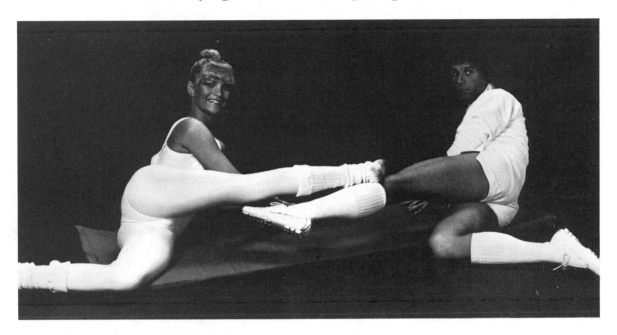

1. Bend underneath legs back.

2. Lift front legs up and out to touch each other.

3. Alternate sides.

CO10 Couples Side Stretch

Position: standing, side to side.

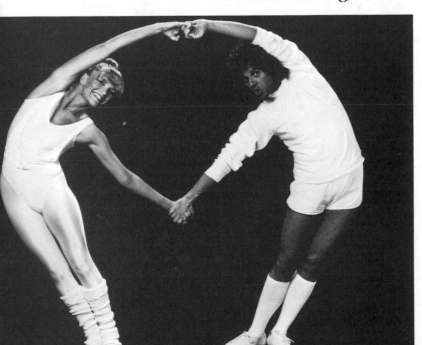

1. Hold both hands and keep feet together.

2. Lean away from each other as you each do a side stretch.

3. Keep your shoulders back.

Menstrual Program

About a week before your period, do you experience lower backache, cramps, fatigue, or moodiness? Believe it or not, exercise can help relieve most of these problems. You get cramps because right before your period a hormonelike substance causes uterine contractions. Some women have more of these hormones released than others, hence they have more severe cramps. Also, while you're having a contraction blood circulation is slower, so nerve endings are more sensitive and you have even more pain. A warm bath, a heating pad, and some stretching exercises will all help the circulation and ease the discomfort.

F13 8 times
and reverse

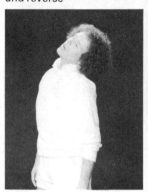

A2 16 times
forward and back

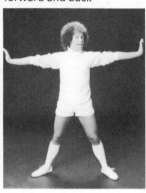

SH7 8
counts hold

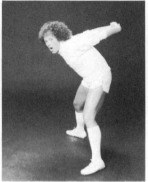

HT1 8 times

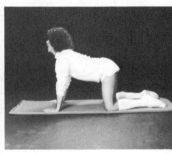

B6 8
counts hold

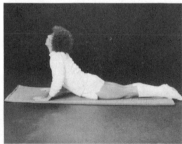

HT2 16 times

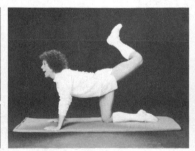

T1 32 times

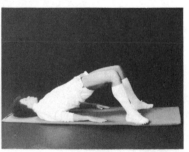

PREGNANCY PROGRAM

Pregnancy causes a tremendous number of changes in your body. (See, I know a lot about this subject.) To ease the transition from one of you to two of you, you will find that exercise eases tension, builds stronger muscles to help you carry the weight, and gets you in better shape for the big moment when you deliver the baby. Most doctors agree that if you are in good physical shape before you become pregnant, you can continue to exercise throughout the pregnancy.

Demonstrated by Abbe Sargent (now Lauren Sargent's mother)

P1 Reach Up, Stretching

Position: standing.

1. **Bend one knee and stretch to that side as you reach up.**

2. **Alternate sides.**

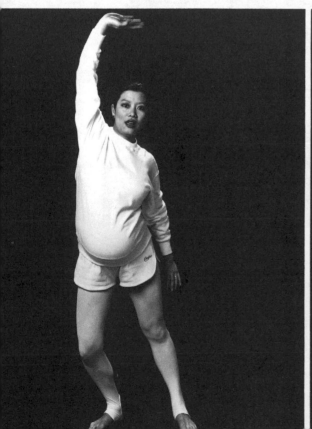
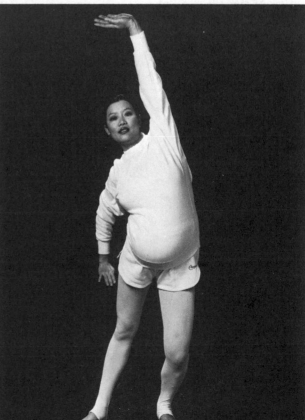

P2 Triangle Pose

Position: standing, arms out to the side.

1. Bend to one side, then lean down and reach overhead at the same time.

2. As you reach up look at your hand.

3. Alternate sides.

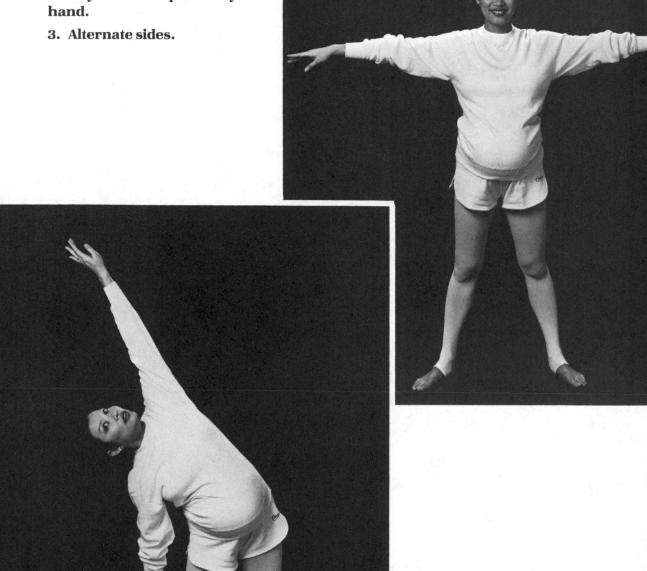

P3 Waist Twist

Position: standing, arms out at your sides.

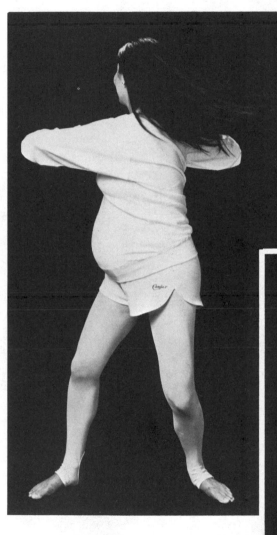

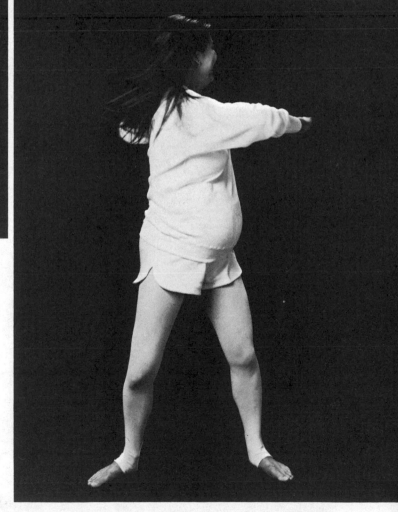

1. **With knees bent, twist at the waist, moving from side to side.**

2. **Don't flail your arms.**

P4 Side to Side

Position: standing, arms out at your sides.

1. Flex your hands, then slide your rib cage from side to side.

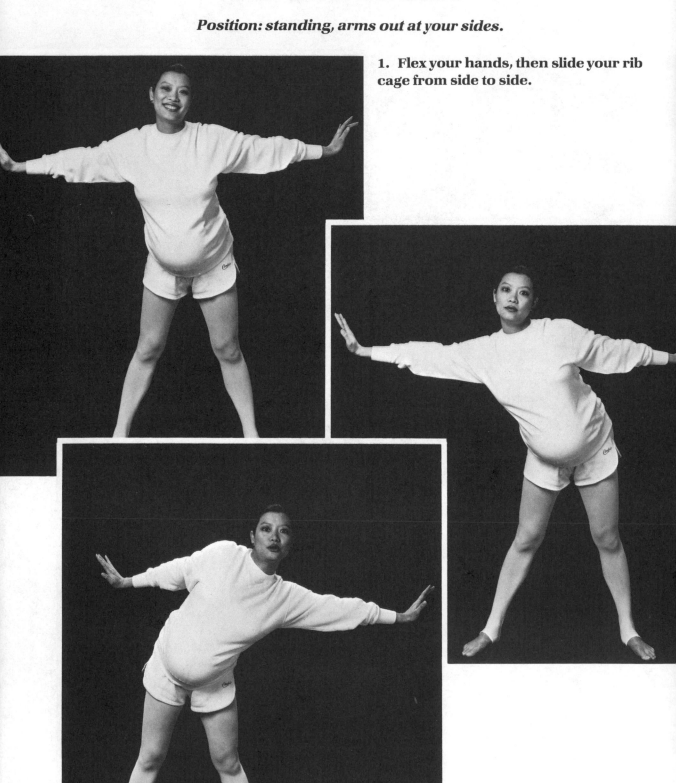

P5 Hip Swings

Position: standing, feet apart.

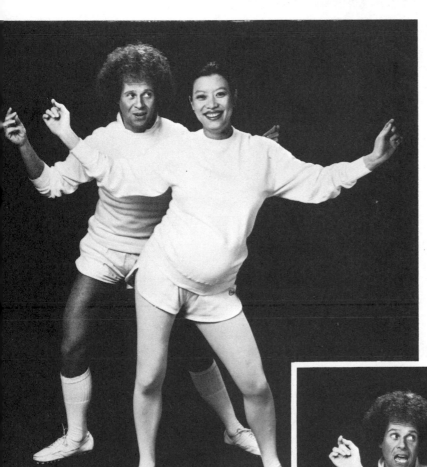

1. **Hold arms up loosely and keep knees bent.**

2. **Rotate your hips smoothly while keeping your shoulders steady.**

3. **This isn't a dance step, so your feet shouldn't move.**

P6 Arm Stretches

Position: standing, feet apart.

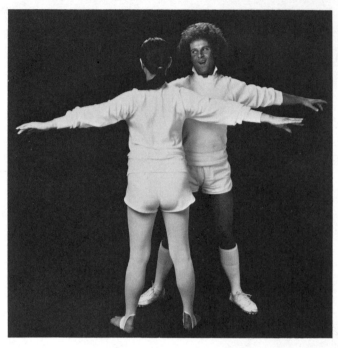

1. Hold your arms out at your sides and pull your shoulder blades back without moving your arms.

2. Keep your head up.

P7 Palm Pushers

Position: standing, feet apart.

1. Hold elbows up and out.

2. Place your fist against your palm and press.

3. Alternate hands.

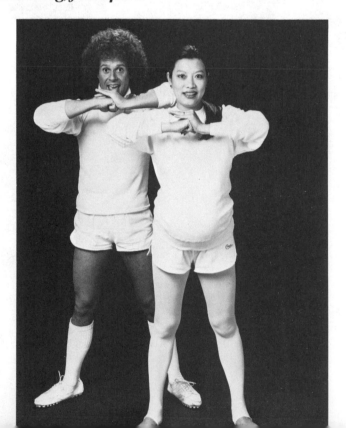

P8 *Flex Fist*

Position: standing, arms out at your sides.

1. Flex hands, then make a fist and repeat.

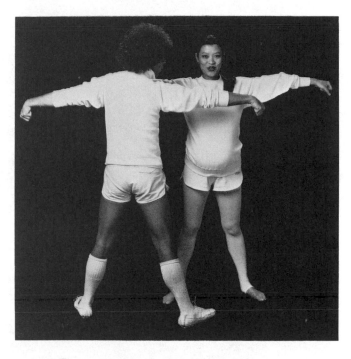

P9 Squats with Legs Apart

Position: standing, feet wide apart, using a straight-back chair for support.

1. Keeping your elbows out and your shoulders up, raise and lower your body.

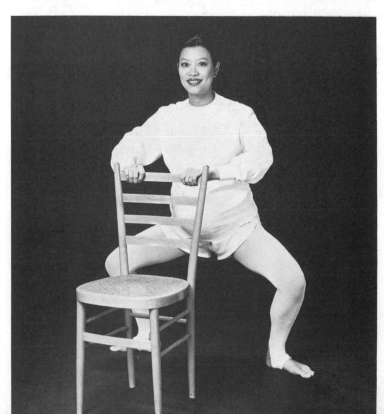

P10 Heel Ups

Position: standing, feet wide apart, using a straight-back chair for support.

1. Keeping your elbow out and your shoulders up, squat with your heels raised off the floor.

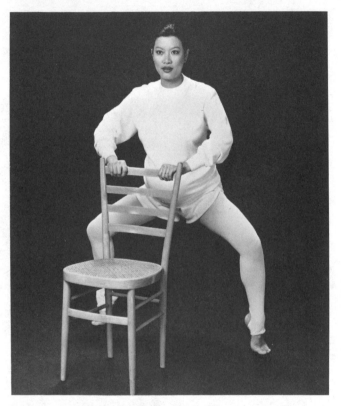

P11 Toe Squats

Position: standing, using a straight-back chair for support.

1. Up on your toes, raise and lower your body without placing heels on the floor.

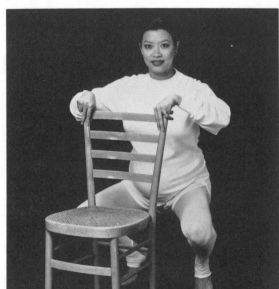

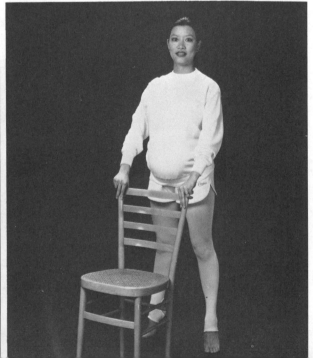

P12 *Back of Leg Stretch*

Position: standing, using a straight-back chair for support.

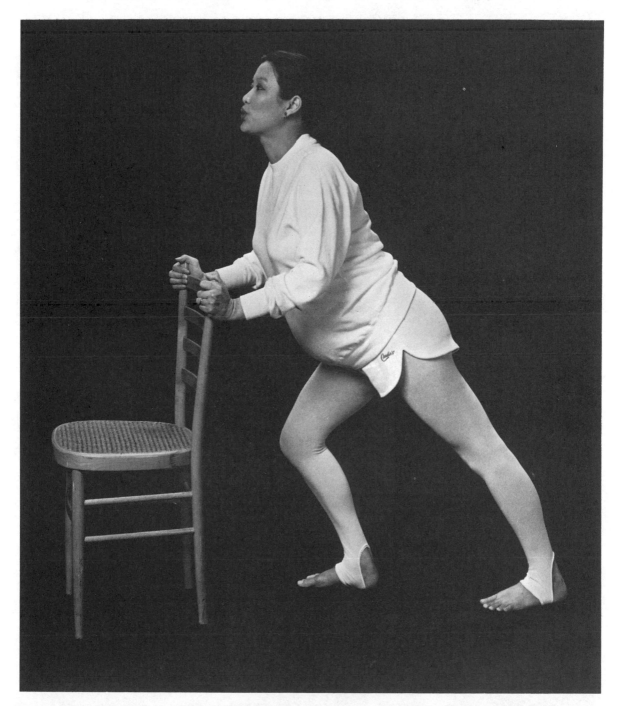

1. **Lean into the chair with one leg forward and one leg back. The forward leg should be bent, and the back leg should be straight.**

2. **Raise yourself up and then lean down again.**

3. **Alternate legs.**

P13 Side Leg Lifts

Position: standing, feet apart, using a straight-back chair for support.

1.   Lean on chair as if it were a ballet bar.

2.   Keeping both legs straight and your feet flexed, raise and lower your leg, never allowing it to quite touch the floor.

3.   Alternate legs.

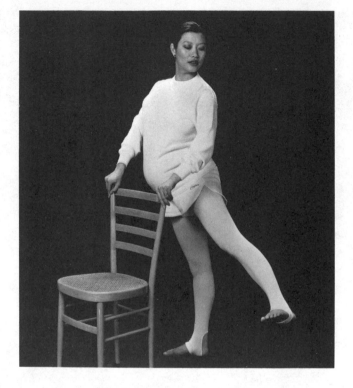

P14 Back Leg Lifts

Position: standing, feet apart, using a straight-back chair for support.

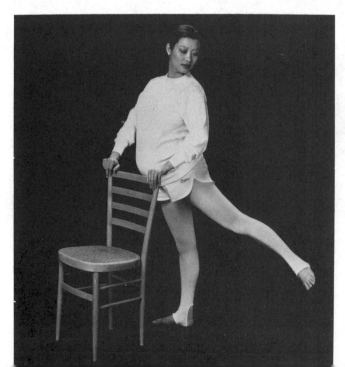

1.   Lean on chair as if it were a ballet bar.

2.   Keeping both legs straight and feet flexed, lift leg back, then raise and lower it, never allowing it to quite touch the floor.

3.   Alternate legs.

P15 *Pregnant Cat Stretch*

Position: on mat, on hands and knees.

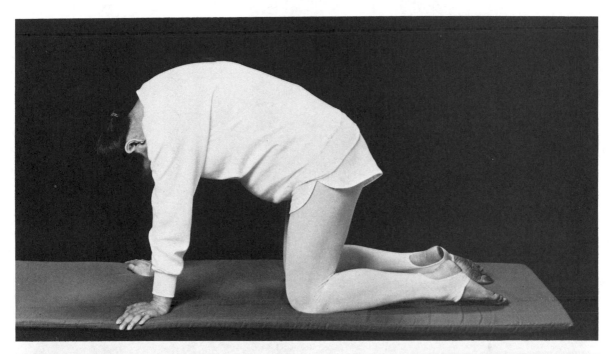

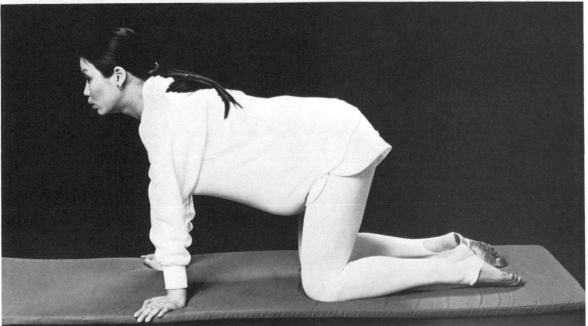

1. Inhale and exhale. Round your back as you inhale, flatten your back as you exhale.

2. Round, flatten, etc.

P16 Pelvic Stretches

Position: on mat, on hands and knees.

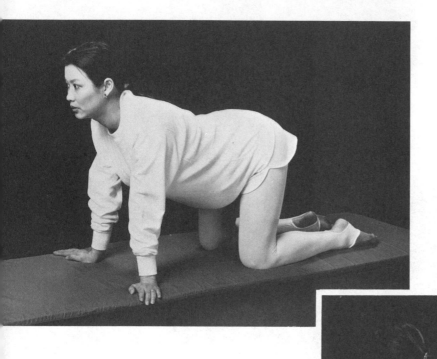

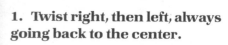

1. Twist right, then left, always going back to the center.

2. Inhale at the center and exhale as you twist your head toward your hip, so you feel the stretch.

P17 Doggy Lifts

Position: on mat, on hands and knees.

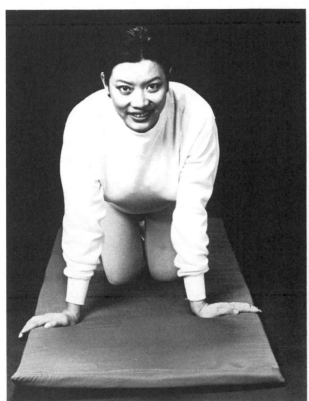

1. Keeping right leg bent, lift it to the side, then put it down.

2. Alternate sides.

3. You should feel this in your tush.

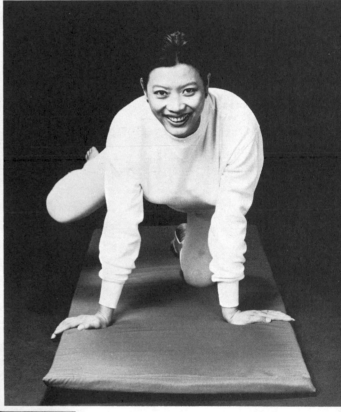

P18 Stretch to Sides

Position: sitting on mat.

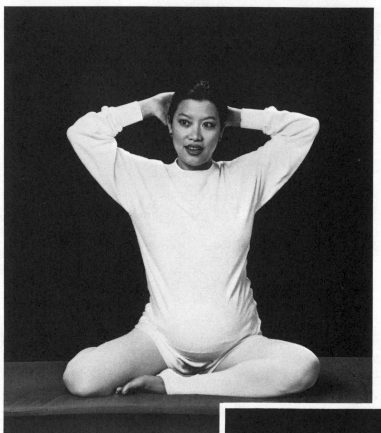

1. Bend one leg behind you, the other in front.

2. Place hands behind your head and stretch, reaching from side to side.

3. Alternate position of legs.

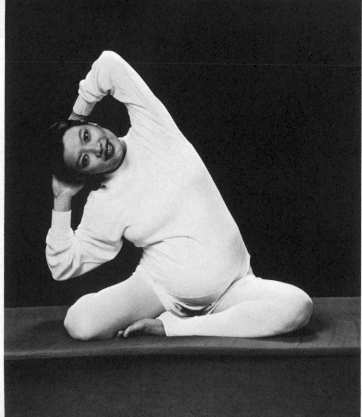

P19 Overhead Stretch

Position: sitting on mat, back straight.

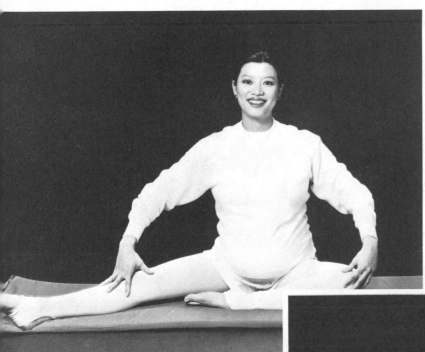

1. **Bend one leg in, stretch the other out to the side.**

2. **Reach over your head to the extended leg.**

3. **Alternate sides.**

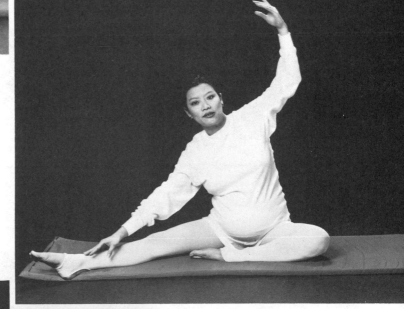

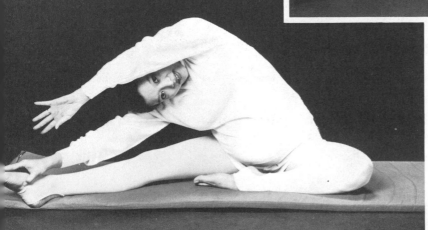

P20 Pregnant Pancake

Position: sitting on mat, legs in straddle position.

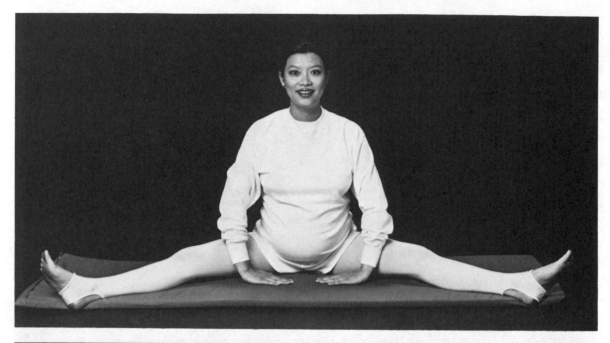

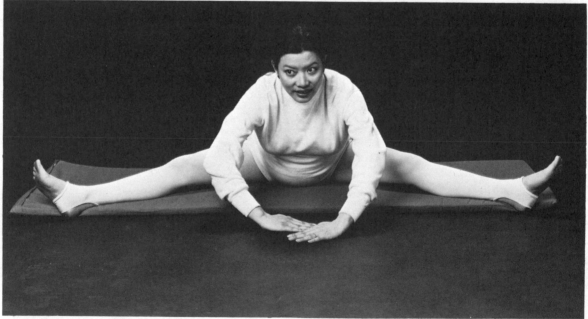

1. When you aren't pregnant, you do a pancake by leaning forward and trying to touch your nose to the floor in front of you.

2. Sitting up tall, supported on your hands, try to get your nose as close to the ground as your belly will allow.

P21 Spinal Twist Straddle Position

Position: sitting on mat, legs in straddle position.

1. Twist from side to side with stops in the center.

2. Take it slow and easy. Don't make the baby seasick.

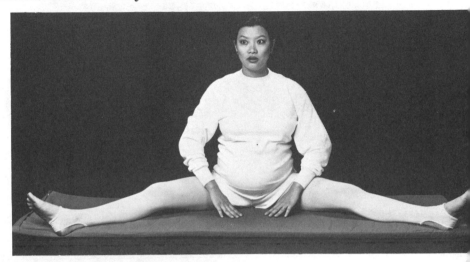

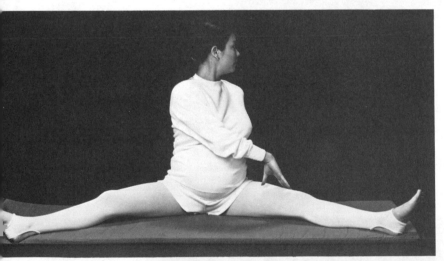

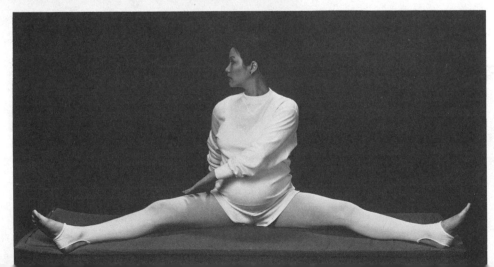

P22 Tootsie Rolls/Buttocks Walk

Position: sitting on mat, legs straight out in front of you.

1. With your hands at your sides, shift your weight from one half of your buttocks to the other.

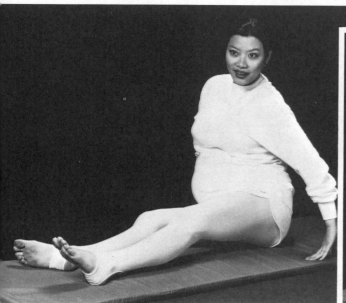
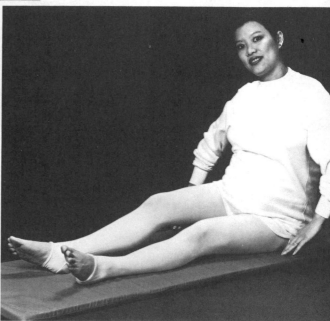

P23 Abdominal Breathing

Position: sitting on mat, knees bent.

1. Round your neck as you exhale. Lift up when you inhale.

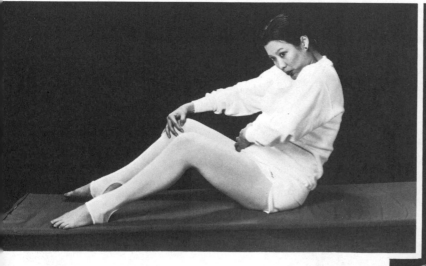
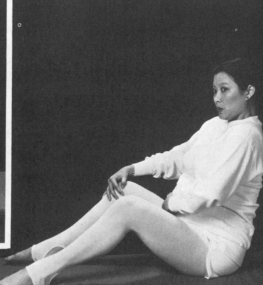

P24 Buttocks Lifts

Position: lying on mat, knees apart and bent.

1. Lift your buttocks up slightly and push spine into the mat.

2. Lower, raise, lower, etc.

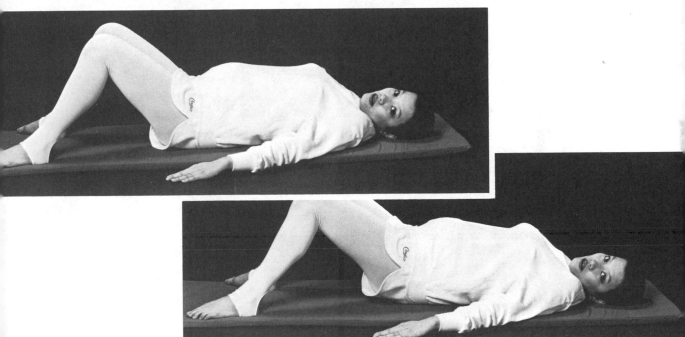

P25 Mini Sit-Ups

Position: lying on mat, knees bent.

1. Just raise your shoulders off the ground, then lower them.

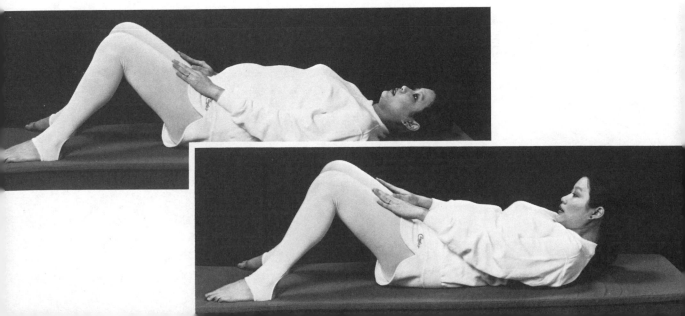

P26 Leg Lifts

Position: lying on mat, legs out straight.

1. With arms down and shoulders rounded, lift one leg at a time.

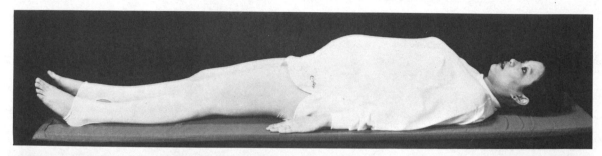

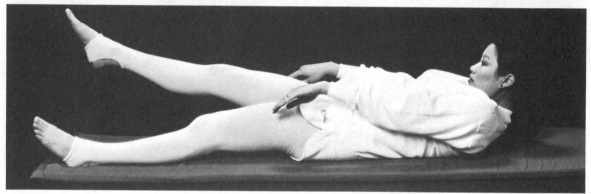

P27 Ankle Rotations

Position: lying on mat, legs out straight.

1. Pull your knee into your belly, then straighten your leg and rotate your ankle. Lower it.

2. Alternate legs.

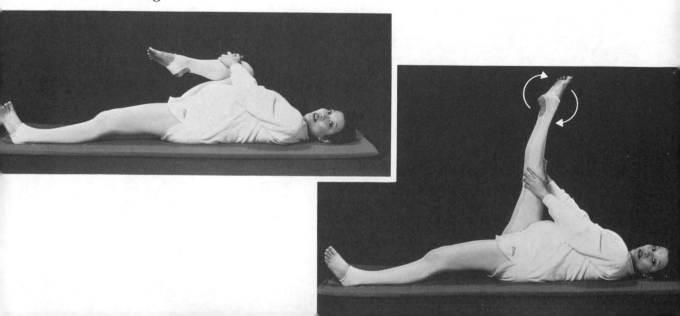

P28 Torso Rolls

Position: sitting cross-legged on mat.

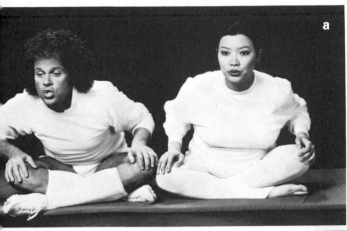

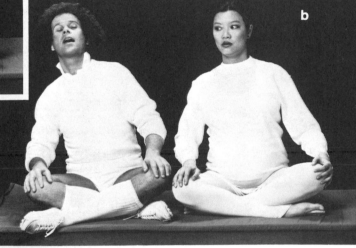

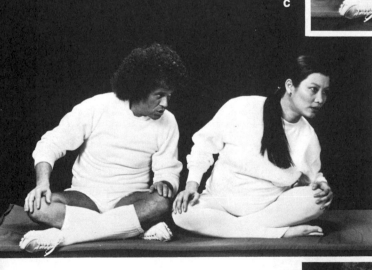

1. With hands on your knees, roll your torso around gently.

P29 Head Rolls

Position: sitting on mat, cross-legged.

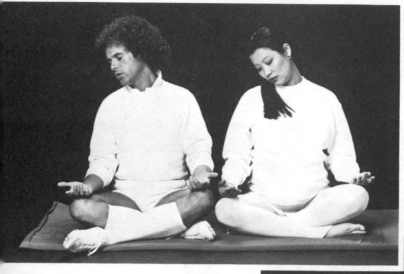

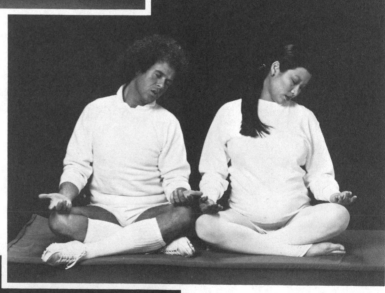

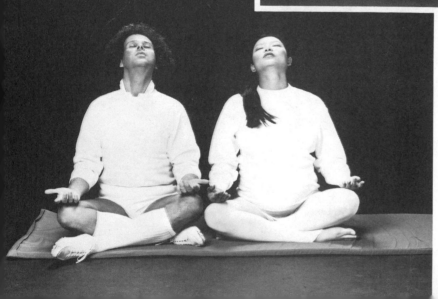

1. Relax your arms, then roll your head around for relaxation.

STRETCH PROGRAM

Stretching is one of those things that cats are really great at and people never quite master. So move over, Garfield, I've got some lessons to give. The stretch program on the following pages is not a plan for beginners (unless you are a cat). It's rather advanced, and if you haven't been exercising regularly the last couple of months (okay, years), you would do well to shape up a little in my BEGINNER plan first (see page 235). But remember this: Stretching is the missing link that connects no activity to maximum activity, and once you're a little looser, you're going to love this program. (The BEGINNER warm-up has some stretching in it—the type of stretching you need to start out with first.)

All warm-up programs begin with some stretching because it's essential that your muscles be ready to do the work you ask of them. This program is a lot more than a big warm-up and it does use every part of the body. It's a great plan for those over fifty and those who are pregnant, handicapped, or not very athletically inclined. But remember, never force a stretch, and if this program hurts, limber up in BEGINNER first.

Stretching is ideal because it keeps the muscles supple and makes the body more flexible. Stretched and relaxed muscles don't pull, sprain, or tear. You'll have fewer injuries (especially if you are a weekend jock) if you use this stretch program before you play any sports. You'll also find that a good stretch session helps to relax your entire being.

While you are stretching, please remember:

- No bouncing, please. Your body is not a basketball. Bouncing can harm the body by tearing the muscle tissue.
- Make sure your body is properly aligned as you do the stretches. If you stretch incorrectly, you will harm your body, and that isn't such a good idea. Proper alignment is essential, so get help if you need it or check your body against mine in these pictures.
- Breathe. No reason to hold your breath, you know.
- If you feel pain, STOP.
- Follow your stretch program patiently and consistently. Don't tease the old bod or reach out to a point of pain. Stretch a little farther each and every day. Consistency is what counts. Never reach out in anger or force . . . and the force will be with you.

ST1 Holding Stretch

Position: standing, feet apart.

1. **Grab the top of your wrist with your other hand. Stretch over from one side to the other while pulling on your wrist.**

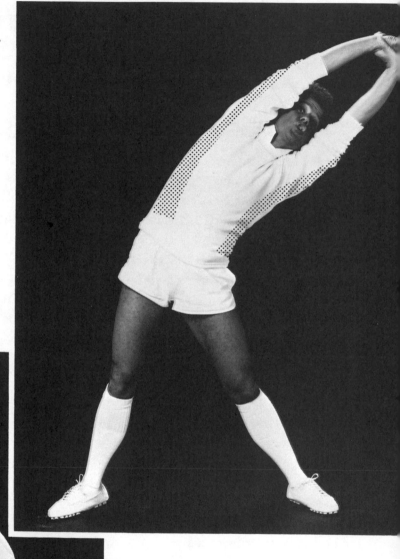

ST2 Triangle Pose

Position: standing, feet apart, arms out to the sides.

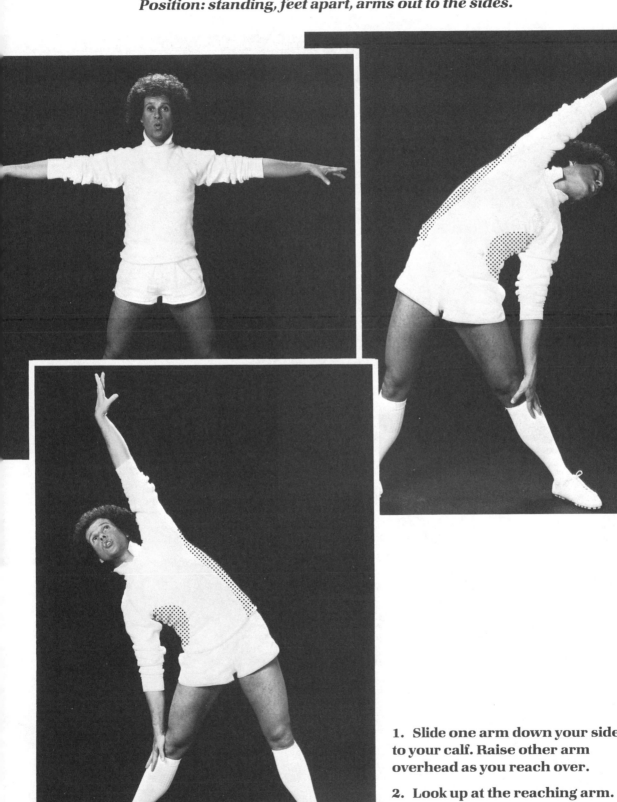

1. Slide one arm down your side to your calf. Raise other arm overhead as you reach over.

2. Look up at the reaching arm.

ST3 Forward Bend Pyramids

Position: standing, feet apart.

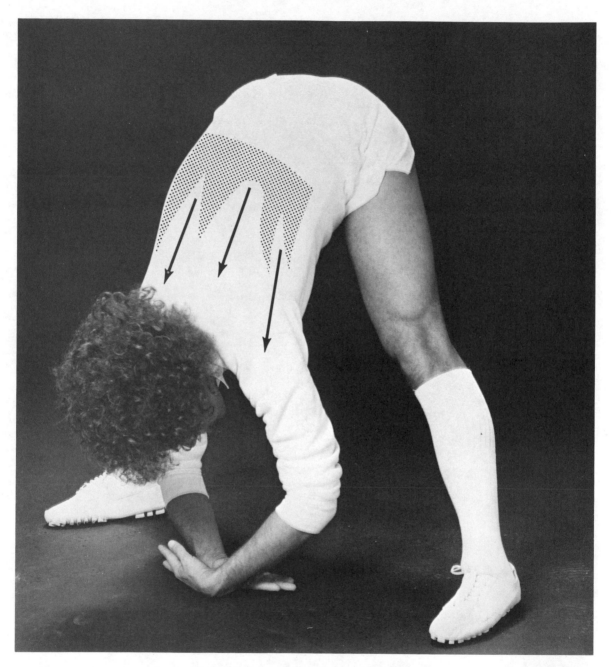

1. Bend over at the waist with your arms clasped and extended in front. Keep your legs straight.

ST4 Holding Toe

Position: standing, feet apart, legs straight.

1. Bend over and hold your toes while you stretch. Don't bounce.

2. Alternate sides.

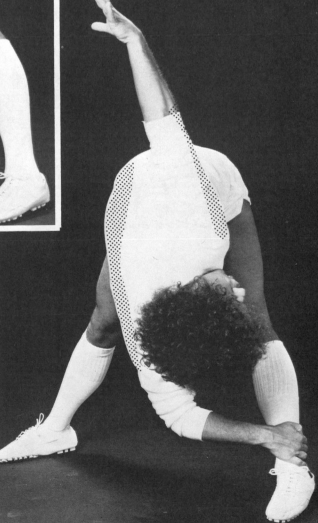

ST5 Forward Bends with Push Throughs

Position: standing, feet apart.

1. Bend forward with knees straight, then with knees bent reach through your legs.

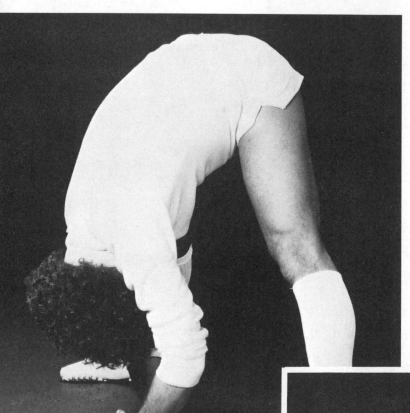

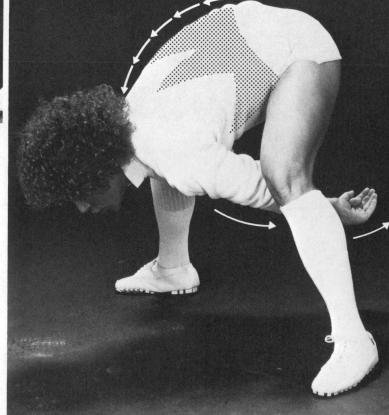

ST6 Holding Profile Lunge

Position: on mat, standing.

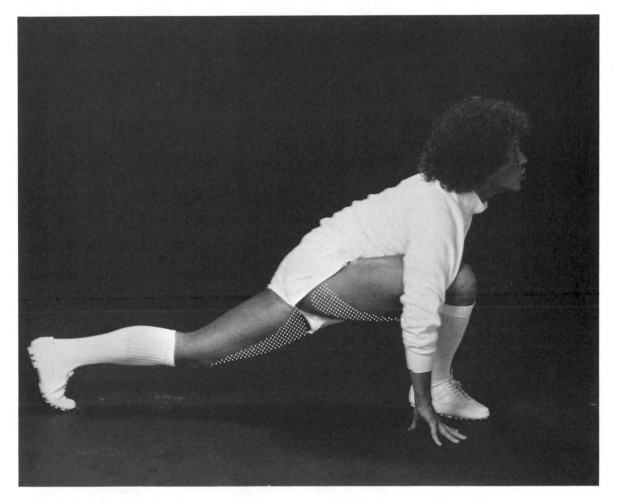

1. **Bending forward, move feet wide apart.**

2. **Place palms down on floor.**

3. **Turn to the right side, bend right leg, and lunge down, keeping left leg straight out behind you.**

4. **Alternate legs.**

ST7 Profile Lunge Up and Down

Position: on mat, standing.

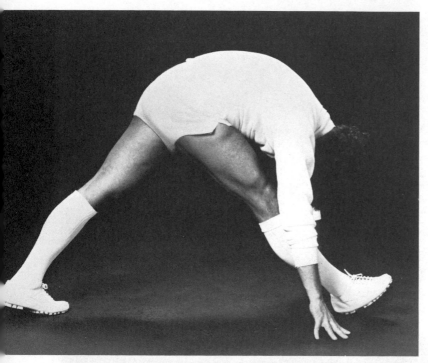

1. Bend over, feet wide apart, with fingers pressed to floor and head down.

2. Bend right leg, lunge forward, then rock back.

3. Alternate legs.

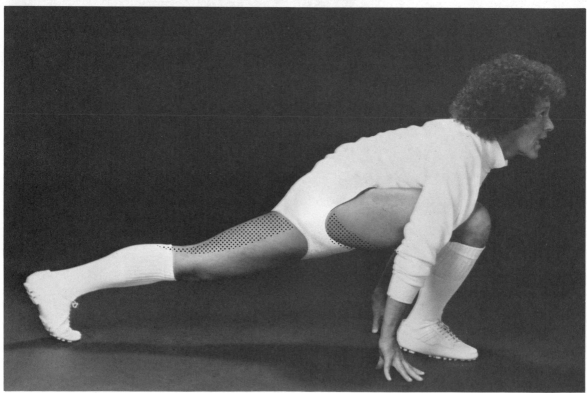

ST8 *Holding Side Stretch*

Position: standing, feet slightly apart, shoulders back.

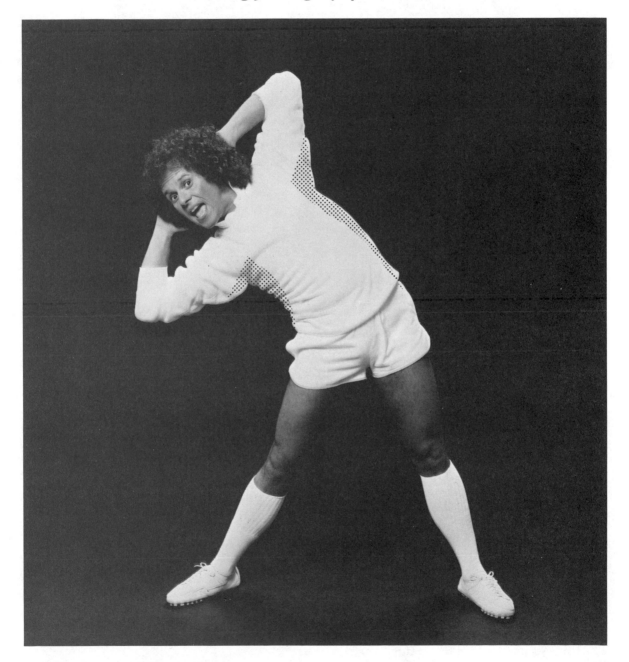

1. **Lace hands behind your head.**

2. **Bend from side to side, holding the stretch, bending only at the waist.**

ST9 Pancake

Position: sitting on mat in straddle position.

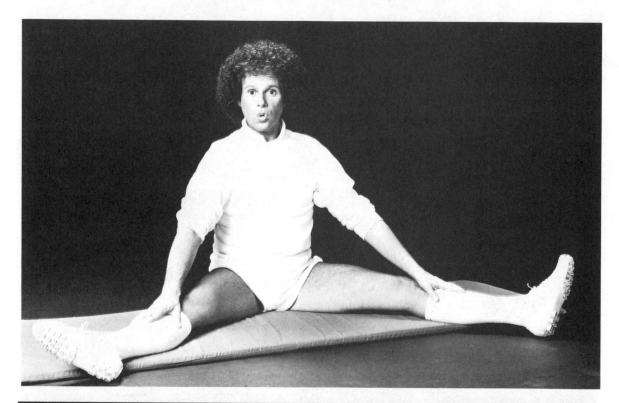

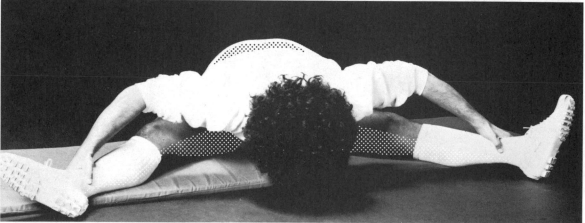

1. Bend forward and try to put your nose on the floor.

ST10 Forward Bends with One Leg Bent

Position: sitting on mat.

1. With one leg straight and one leg bent, lean to the side of the straight leg and stretch over, feeling the pull in your hips.

2. Alternate sides.

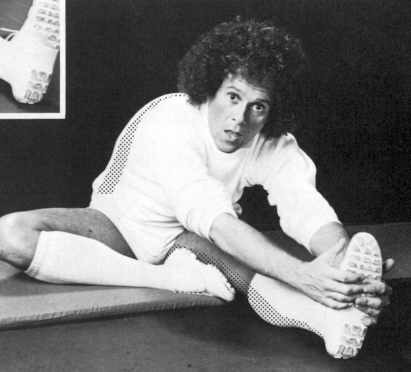

ST11 Forward Bend with Legs Out Front

Position: sitting on mat with legs straight out in front.

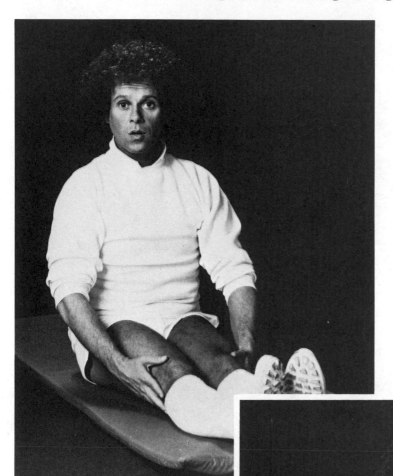

1. Grab your feet with your hands to help pull you into the stretch.

ST12 Forward Bend in Frog Pond

Position: sitting on mat.

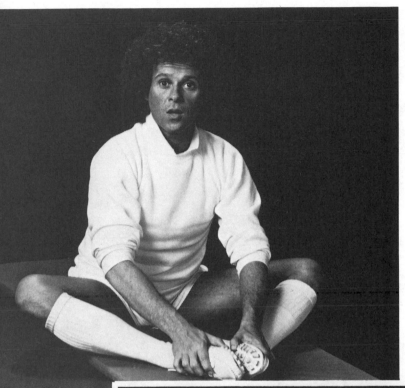

1. With soles of the feet together and knees bent, use your hands to hold your toes as you bend forward.

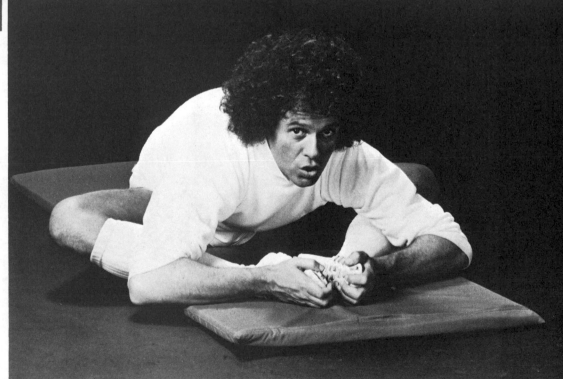

ST13 Side Bend with One Leg Bent

Position: sitting on mat.

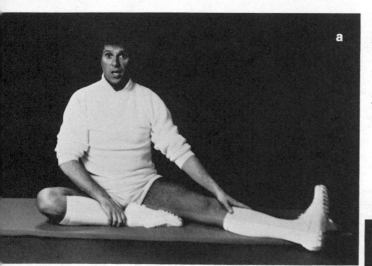

1. With one leg bent and one leg straight out to the side, reach arms overhead toward the ankle of the straight leg.

2. Alternate sides.

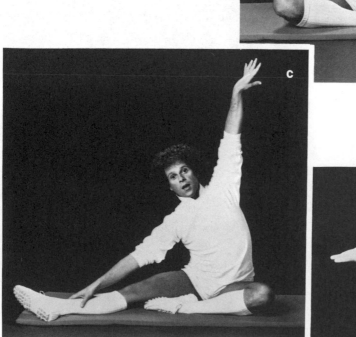

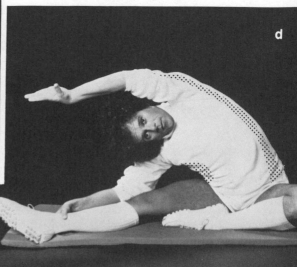

ST14 Forward Bend with One Leg Bent

Position: sitting on mat.

1. With one leg bent and one leg straight out to the side, reach forward.

2. Alternate position of legs.

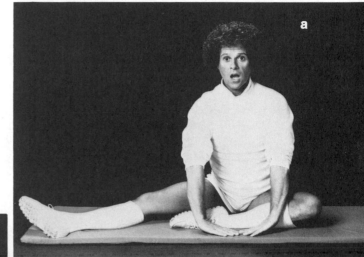

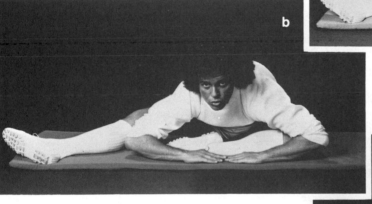

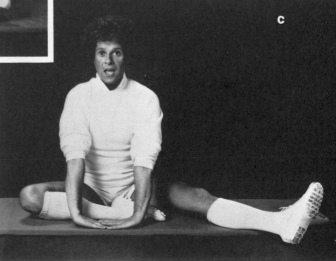

ST15 One Leg Bent Back

Position: sitting on mat.

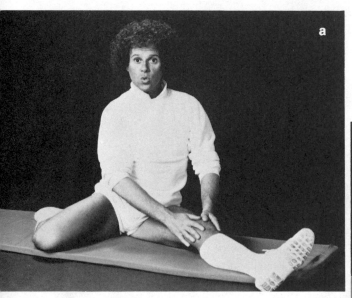

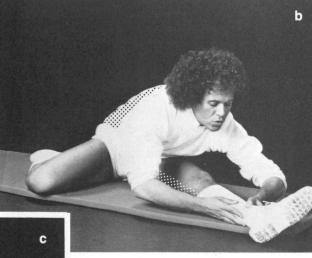

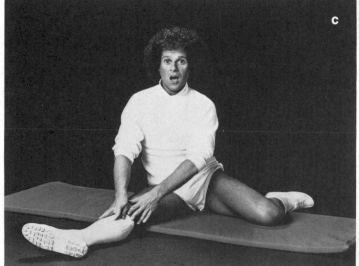

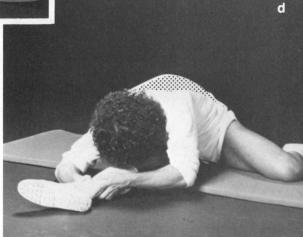

1. With one leg forward and one leg bent back, reach forward.

2. Alternate position of legs.

ST16 Knee Grabs and Ups

Position: lying on mat.

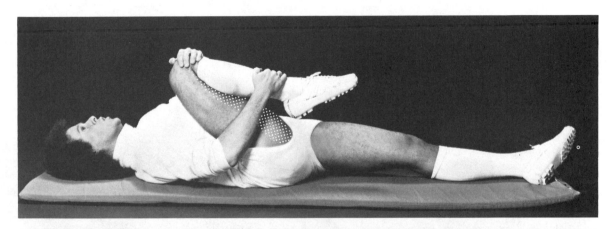

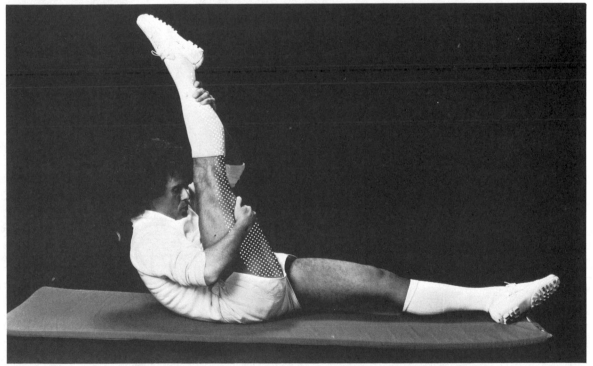

1. Bring leg to your chest in a leg grab, then extend the leg up and forward as close to your face as you can get it.

2. Of course it hurts. Use your hands to pull the leg closer to you.

ST17 Spinal Twist

Position: lying on mat.

1. Bend one leg in with the other leg crisscrossed on top of it.

2. Twist your body in the same direction as the top leg is pointing.

3. Twist your head with your body.

4. Alternate legs.

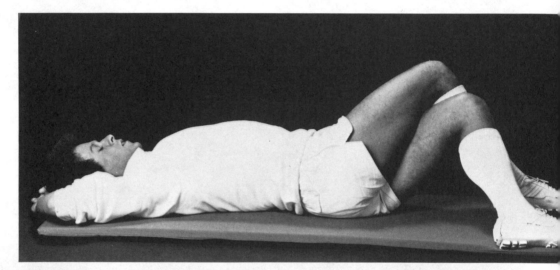

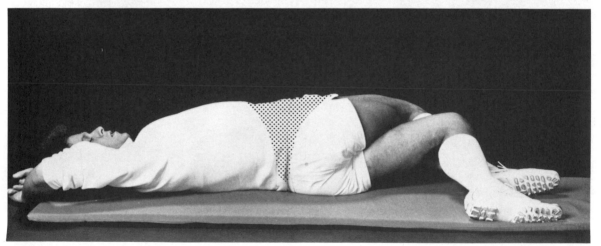

ST18 *Froggy on the Pond*

Position: on mat, lying down.

1. With shoulders and head up, put your feet together and grab them with your hands.

2. Keep knees bent and apart, and use your hands to press your ankles closer to your body while lowering your back.

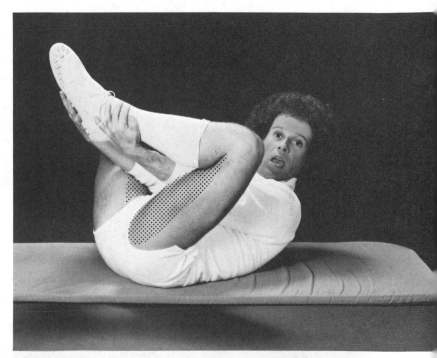

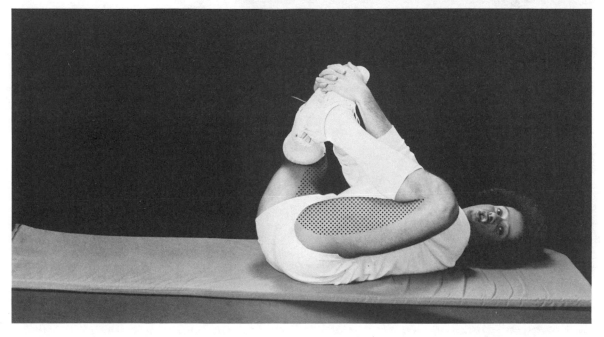

ST19 Cat Stretches

Position: on mat, on hands and knees.

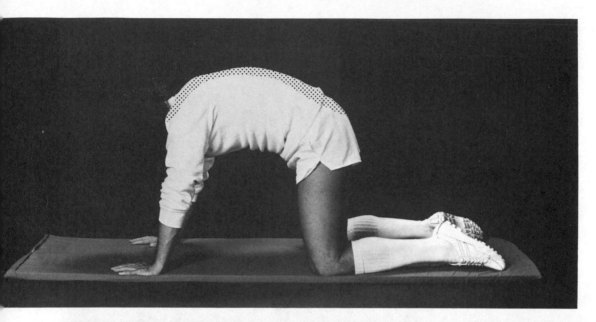

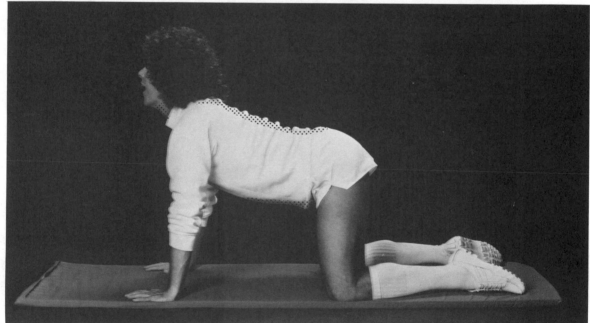

1. **Knees are apart, palms are flat on the ground.**

2. **Lower your head, inhale, arch your back, raise your head, and exhale; then lower your head, inhale, etc.**

ST20 *Pelvic Stretches*

Position: on mat, on hands and knees.

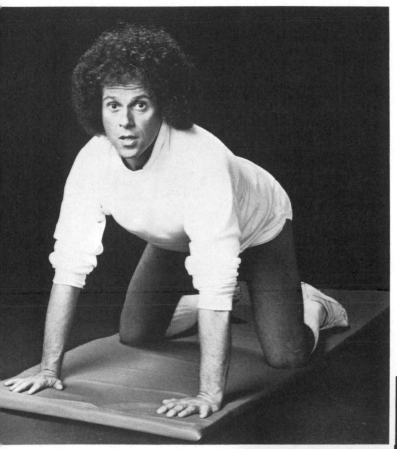

1. Twist right, then left, always going back to the center.

2. Inhale at the center and exhale as you twist your head toward your hip, so you feel the stretch.

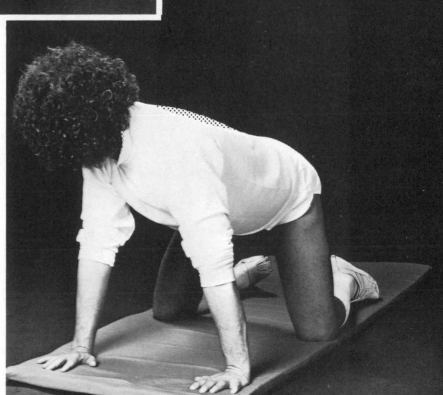

ST21 Cobra

Position: on mat, lying on stomach.

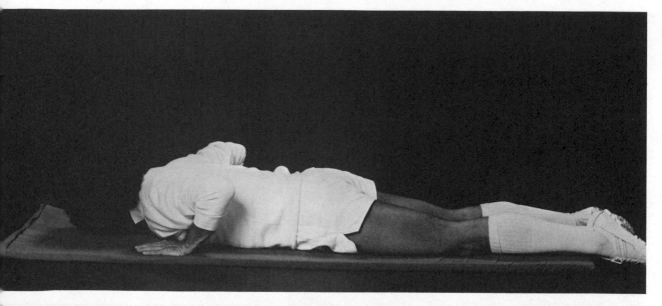

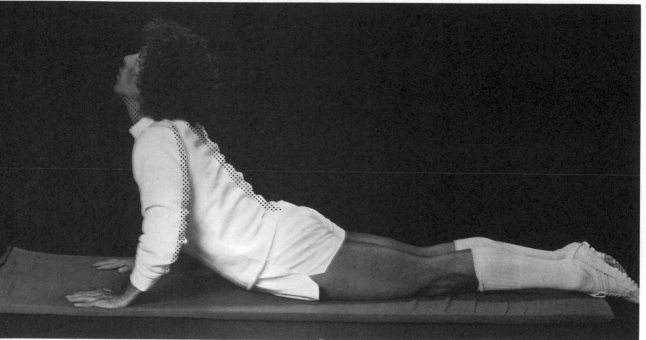

1. Toes are pointed, head is curled back, and palms are flat on the mat with the elbows bent.

2. Pull yourself up and lower yourself down.

ST22 Cobra Twist

Position: on mat, lying on stomach.

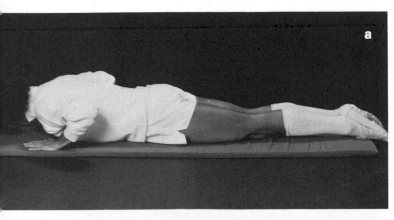

1. Toes are pointed, head is curled back, and palms are flat on the mat with the elbows bent.

2. Take your right arm, put it behind you, and grab your left hip.

3. Make sure your hips stay on the ground.

4. Alternate sides.

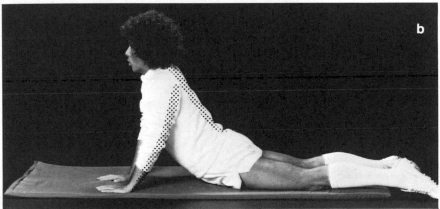

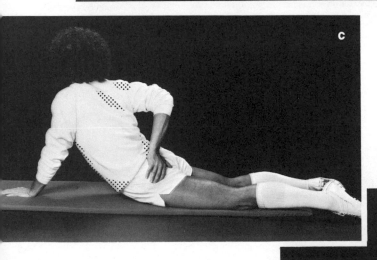

Silver Citizens' Program

Somebody out there thinks that older people will break in two if they attempt to exercise. There are no exercise books for silver citizens, and there are few special classes. Experts on aging seem to encourage basket weaving and clay modeling to keep the fingers moving, but little else. Well, folks, not me. There is no reason for you not to exercise—from infancy to your silver years.

If you have always exercised and used your body, you'll find the aging process is more kind to you and that you are able to do more things easier for a longer period of time. But if you haven't exercised for twenty, thirty, forty, or more years, you can still begin now. You'll need to go slow and it might take you a good while to advance to the BEGINNER program, but you will advance. I have silver citizens in my aerobics class, and they are as fit as I am.

Demonstrated by Sy and Betty Rothkopp

SC1 Chews

(Yes, these are Sy's and Betty's real teeth!)

Position: in front of a mirror.

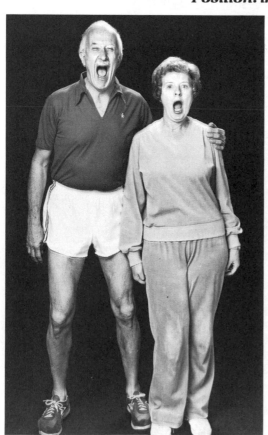

1. **Neck up, smile a big Miss America smile.**

2. **Chew the air without grinding your teeth.**

SC2 Side Wipes

Position: in front of a mirror.

1. Contort your face in a pout first to the left, then to the right.

2. It's not unusual for one side to be easier than the other.

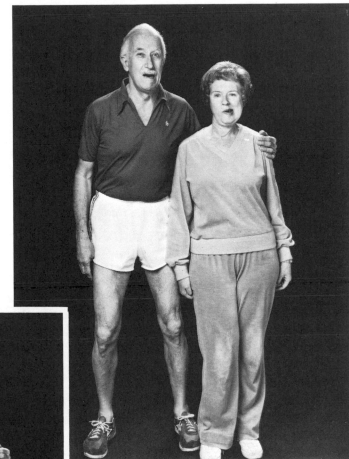

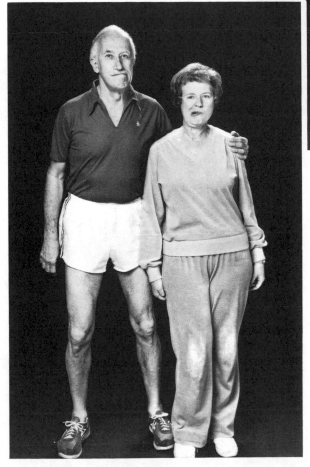

SC3 Neck Forward and Back Stretch, Then Up and Down

Position: standing, shoulders back, neck straight.

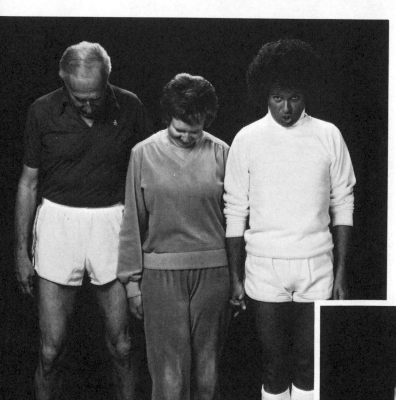

1. Using your best military posture, stretch your neck forward, touching your chin *almost* to your chest, then stretch your neck backward (without leaning your body back).
2. Do this exercise slowly, stretching out those stiff muscles. Don't jerk your head back and forth too quickly.

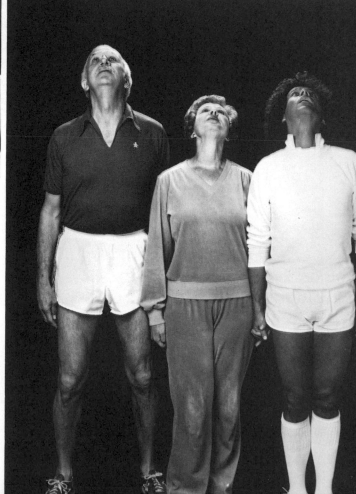

SC4 *Side to Side, Ear to Shoulder*

Position: standing, shoulders back, neck held high

1. Plant your feet slightly apart and stretch your neck first to the left, then to the right.
2. Don't bring your shoulders up to meet your neck when you do this exercise—that's cheating!

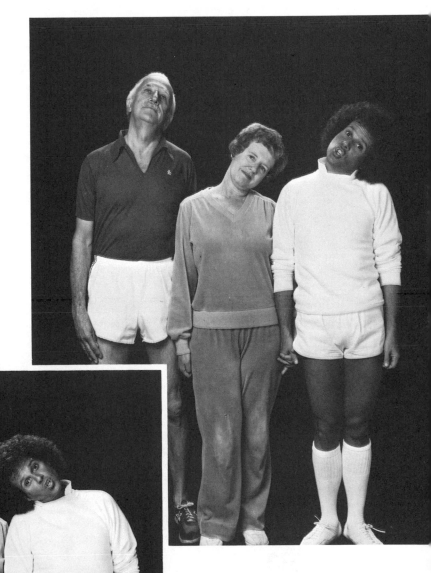

SC5 Shoulder Shrugs, Up and Down, Hands Flexed

Position: standing, feet slightly apart.

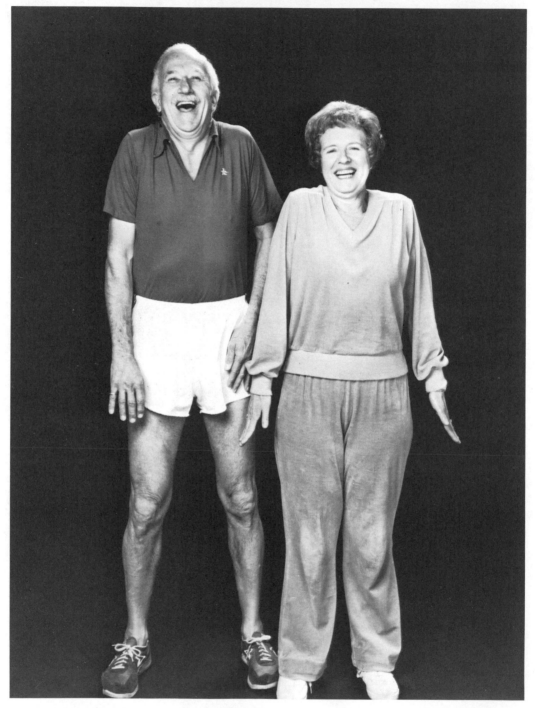

1. Lift your shoulders up to your ears while keeping your back straight.

2. Drop your shoulders down to their regular position.

SC6 *Shoulders Forward and Back*

Position: standing, feet slightly apart.

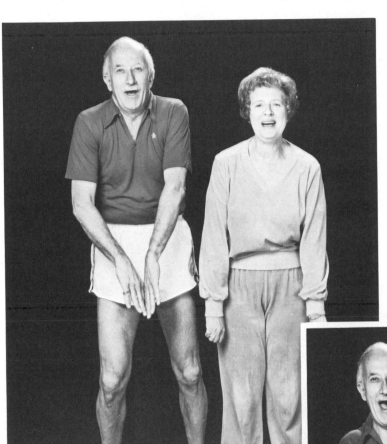

1. Move your shoulders forward while keeping your back up and straight, then bring them back.

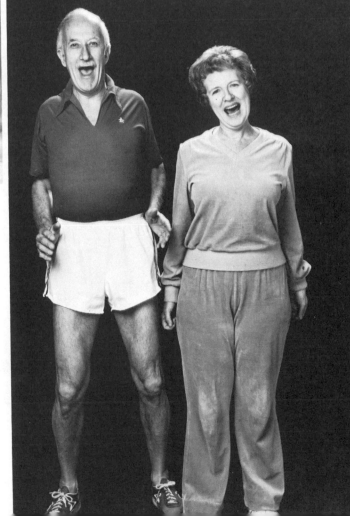

SC7 Reach Overhead and Hold, Then Alternate Sides

Position: standing, feet slightly apart.

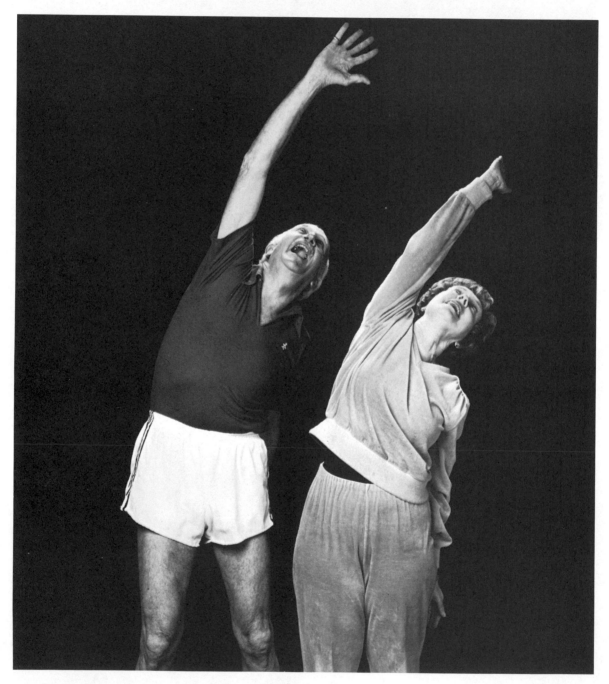

1. **Bend right knee and reach up with right arm.**
2. **Lean into the reach, arching your arm overhead.**
3. **Alternate sides.**

SC8 Side Crawls, Down

Position: standing, feet slightly apart, back straight.

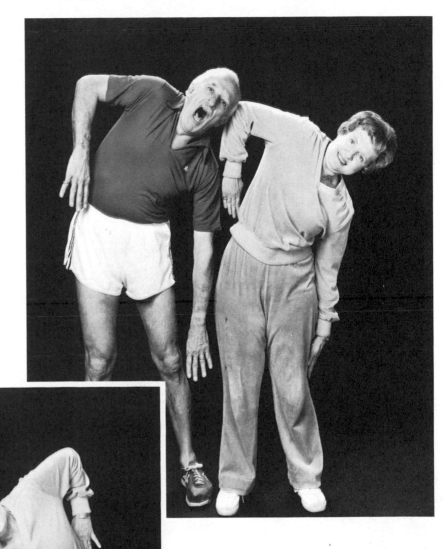

1. Lean to the left while you keep your hips tight and straight, so that you bend only at the waist.
2. Alternate sides.

SC9 Running in Place

Position: standing, shoulders back.

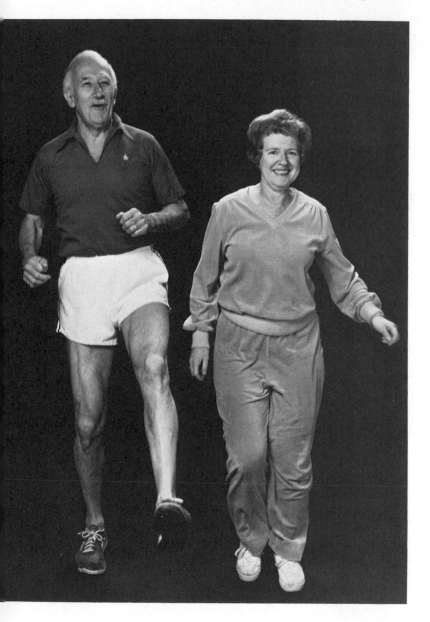

1. Making sure that your heels touch the ground, run in place, 5–10 minutes.

SC10 *Skips in Front*

Position: standing, shoulders back.

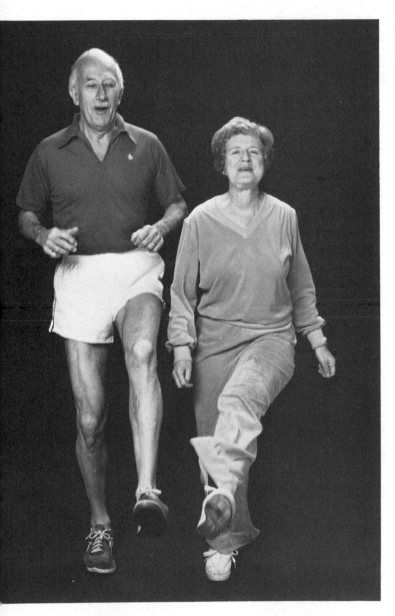

1. Skip your legs out in front of you without really going anywhere.

SC11 Arm Hugs

Position: standing, feet slightly apart.

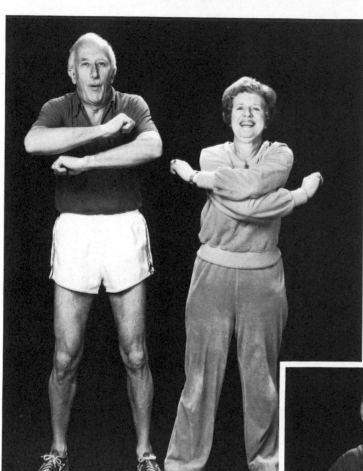

1. Give yourself a hug, crossing your bent arms in front of you, with your hands in fists.
2. Change arms from front to back as you cross and uncross.
3. You should feel this in your upper back.

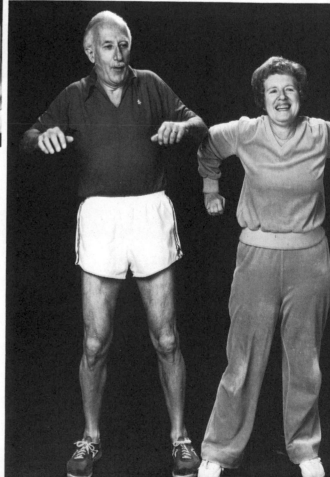

SC12 Lifts on Back with Knees Together and Bent, Feet Apart, Hands Behind Head

Position: on mat, lying on back, knees bent.

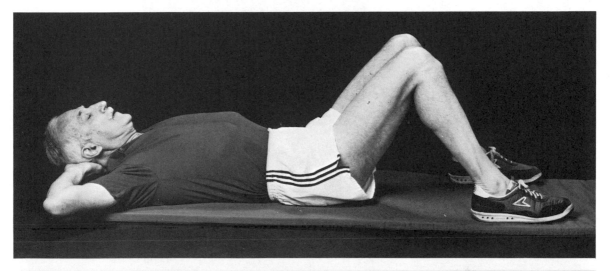

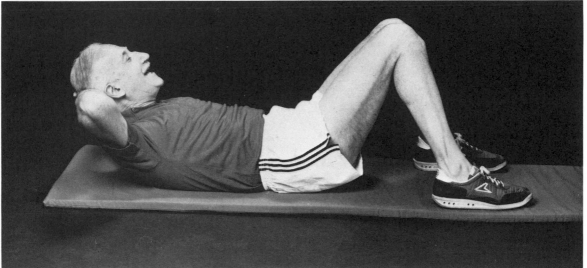

1. Slowly lift yourself up from the waist, bringing your shoulders off the mat. Keep your elbows locked into position.

2. Slowly lower yourself to the mat.

SC13 Reach Between Legs—Lying Down Reaches

Position: on mat, lying down, legs apart.

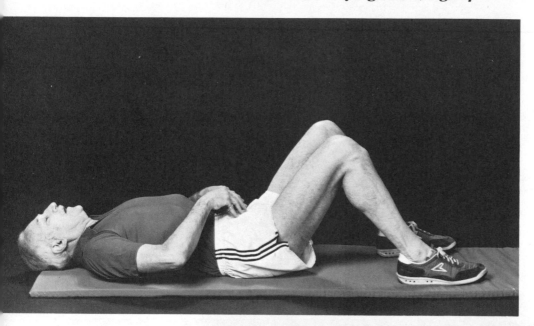

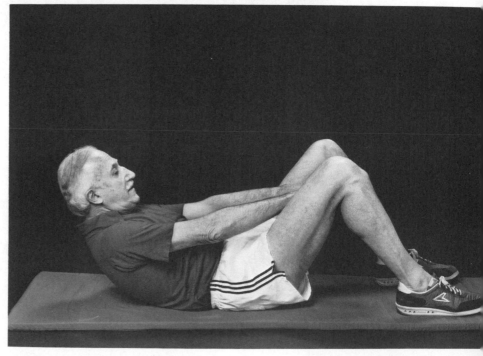

1. With your feet on the floor and your knees bent, sit up and reach through your legs, bouncing back and forth.

SC14 Froggy on the Pond

Position: on mat, lying down.

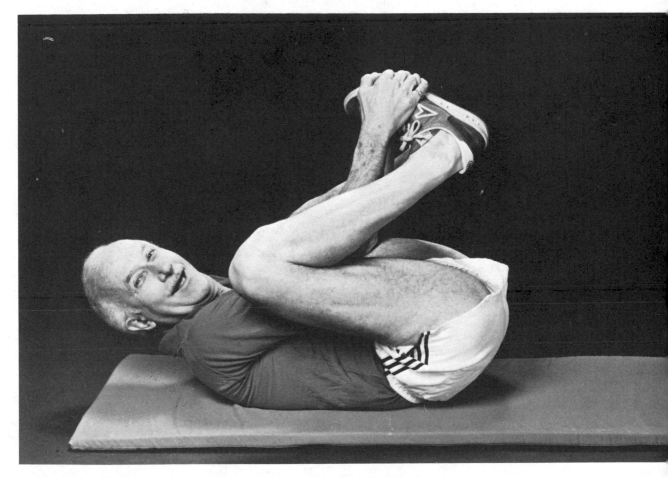

1. With shoulders and head up, put your feet together and grab them with your hands.

2. Keep knees bent and apart and use your hands to press your ankles closer to your body while lowering your back.

SC15 Cobra

Position: on mat, lying on stomach.

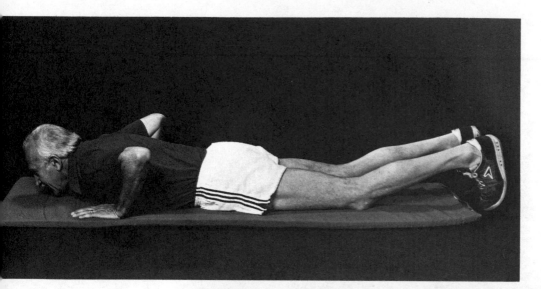

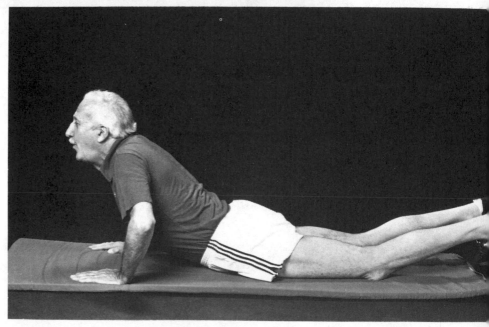

1. Toes are pointed, head is curled back, and palms are flat on the mat with the elbows bent.

2. Pull yourself up and lower yourself down.

SC16 Minilifts

Position: on mat, lying on back, hands at your sides.

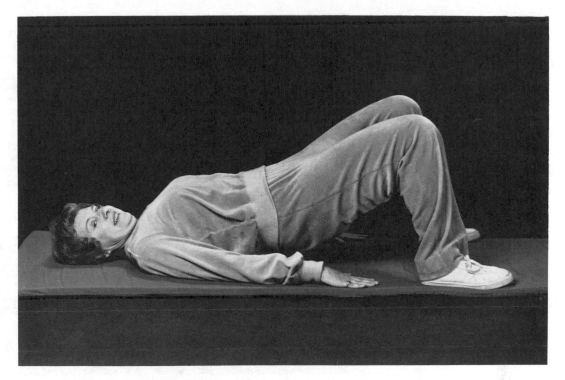

1. With knees bent, slowly lift your back off the mat.
2. Slowly lower yourself to the mat.

SC17 Doggy Lifts

Position: on mat, on hands and knees.

1. Keeping right leg bent, lift it to the side, then put it down.

2. Alternate legs.

3. You should also feel this in your tush.

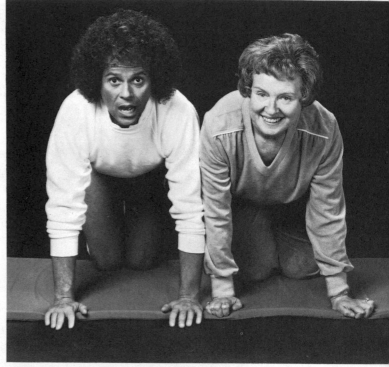

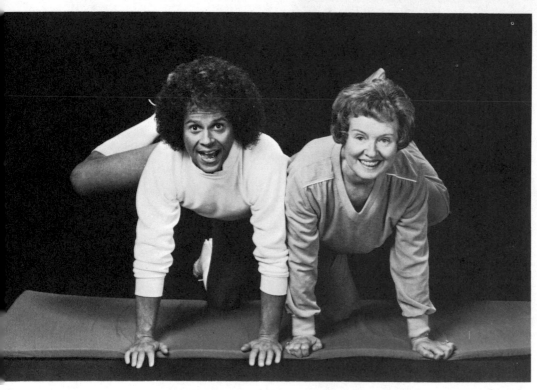

SC18 Leg Lifts

Position: on mat, lying on side, supported by one elbow.

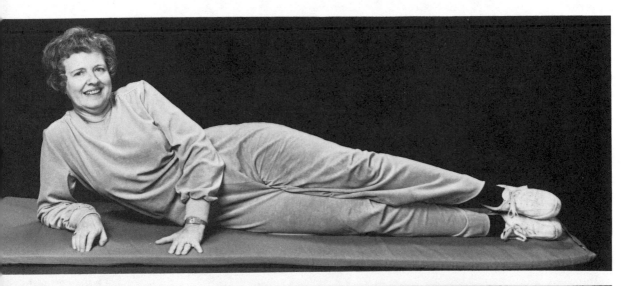

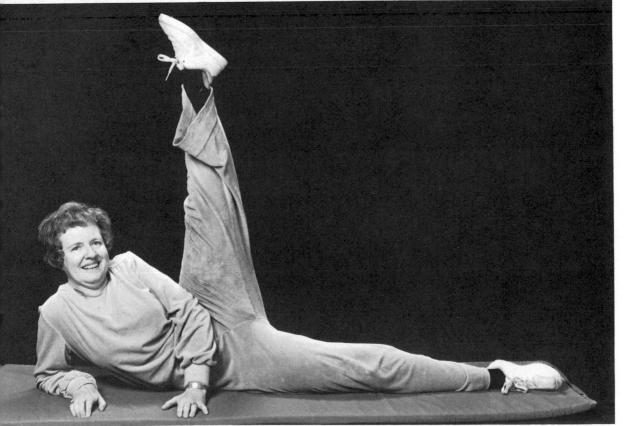

1. Keep your chest up and your abdomen in.

2. Lift left leg up while flexed at ankle so heel is higher than toes. Keep hip forward, and don't worry about raising it up too high—it's impossible.

3. Alternate legs.

Never-Say-You-Can't-Win-a-Contest
Contest Winners

Well, the Richard Simmons Never-Say-You-Can't-Win-a-Contest Contest is finally over, and six people will never again say that they can't win a contest. The six winners (and one guest of their choice) were flown to Los Angeles, and a good time was had by all.

The winners stayed at a posh Beverly Hills hotel (after being picked up at the airport in a snazzy limousine). They were treated to facials at a famous beauty spot in Beverly Hills, cocktails at a well-known clothing establishment frequented by celebrities, dinners at two of the more famous restaurants in town, a day at the magic kingdom of Disneyland, and parties.

So many people helped to make this weekend a great success, and I would like to thank:

- Amy Walters at Wamsutta Mills
- Steve Blunck at Balloon Bouquets
- Bob Roth at Disneyland
- Kathryn Klinger at Georgette Klinger salon
- Fred Hayman at Giorgio
- Patrick Terrail at Ma Maison
- Gerard Ferry and Nicole Winkler at Pastel Cafe
- Sheila Mack (and all her helpers)
- Judith Thomas at Panache Interiors.

The dinners we had during the L.A. weekend were particularly successful, and everyone loved the low-calorie food so much that I mailed them the recipes and thought that you might like to have them, too.

From the Kitchen of Pastel Cafe

PASTEL CHICKEN

> 1 roasting chicken
>   seasonings

If the weather is warm enough, use the rotisserie on your barbecue for this chicken. If not, use a standing chicken rack. This way your chicken stands up and all the fat will drip off.
- *Inside the chicken:* Put onion, shallot, garlic, parsley, thyme, rosemary, sage, pepper, and salt substitute.
- *Outside the chicken:* Put salt substitute, pepper, thyme, and garlic powder.
- Roast until golden brown.

STEAMED PARSLEY

- Cut off the stems and steam!

FLOATING PINEAPPLE YUM-YUM

> 2 eggs
>   dash of sugar
>
> ½ a fresh pineapple
>   strawberries for garnish

- Puree fruit of the pineapple.
- Separate eggs, using only the whites. Beat until they form peaks, adding small amounts of sugar to help stiffen.
- Poach egg whites in two mounds or cook in bain-marie in two molds until firm.
- Divide pureed pineapple into two parts, putting each half in a crystal bowl or a wide champagne glass. Top with meringue and garnish with strawberries.
- Yield: two servings.

From the Kitchen of Ma Maison

GRILLED SALMON

6 oz. salmon per person
tomatoes, peeled, seeded, diced
shallots, minced

lime juice
olive oil
mint, chopped

- Mix tomatoes, shallots, lime juice, and mint together, slowly adding just enough olive oil to moisten.
- Broil salmon until cooked
- Place grilled salmon on bed of mixture.
- Serve immediately.

MA MAISON SALAD

red leaf lettuce
endive
avocado

pine nuts, roasted
scallops

- Place lettuce on plate. On top of lettuce place endive, sliced avocado, pine nuts, and scallops.
- Serve with a vinaigrette dressing.

POACHED PEARS

juice of ½ lemon
juice of ½ lime
1 tsp. vanilla extract

equal parts sugar and water
2 tbsp. honey
½ pear per person

- Place all ingredients in a saucepan. Bring to a boil.
- Add pears. Cook until pears are tender (five to twenty minutes, depending on the size and ripeness of pears).
- Cover with water. Add honey.

The Winners

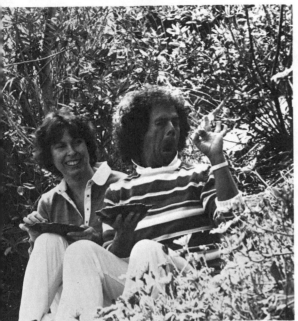

Margaret Thompson
FAMILY PICNIC

Ever since I was six years old my family has been vacationing in the Adirondack Mountains in New York. As we all grew up (I have two sisters and a brother) vacation time became one of the times in the year when we could all come together with my parents and have a little fun. Recently my father and mother bought a cottage at Saranac Lake, and we all gather there periodically and talk and cook ourselves silly! I now have four children of my own, and my sisters are married, so we have quite a crowd! When I read about this contest, it became a challenge for me to devise a menu that wouldn't do too much damage to the waistline! What better group to try it on than my own family! Not only was it challenging in the low-cal aspect but, as you might surmise, our accommodations are not deluxe and there are not all the comforts of my own kitchen. Things took a lot longer to do, but everything can be prepared a day in advance. The meal can be eaten either hot or cold and is portable.

⊷ MENU ⊶

Raw Vegetables with Cucumber Yogurt Dip
Rolled Chicken with Spinach Ricotta Spiral
Stuffed Tomatoes with Zucchini
Green Salad with Mustard Vinaigrette
Assorted Fruits

RAW VEGETABLES WITH CUCUMBER YOGURT DIP

Assorted vegetables: carrots, celery, zucchini, cucumbers, green beans, green peppers, all washed and sliced
  1 red pepper, washed and seeds scooped out

1 cucumber, squeezed dry and shredded
1 large container low-fat plain yogurt
  basil
  black pepper, to taste

- Mix shredded cucumber, yogurt, and seasonings together.
- Spoon dip mixture into center of red pepper. Arrange vegetables around pepper.

ROLLED CHICKEN WITH SPINACH RICOTTA SPIRAL

2 large whole chickens, skinned, boned, and laid flat

- Place chicken on cheesecloth and set aside.

Spinach Ricotta Filling

2 packages frozen chopped spinach, with liq-uid squeezed out
1 lb. skimmed milk ricotta cheese

$\frac{1}{4}$ cup green onion, chopped
1 large clove garlic
black pepper

- Mix all ingredients together and spread evenly on chicken, leaving a border of about half an inch.
- Roll chicken up, using cheesecloth to help you. Wrap cheesecloth around chicken so you have a fairly neat roll, then tie with kitchen string.
- Bake chicken in the oven at 350° F for 1½ hours or until juices run clear when chicken is pierced.
- Let stand till cool enough to handle, then carefully unwrap chicken from cheesecloth and slice.
- Can be served hot or cold.

STUFFED TOMATOES WITH ZUCCHINI

1 dozen tomatoes
2 medium zucchini, grated, with moisture squeezed out
2 tbsp. butter
1 minced clove garlic

black pepper
basil
$\frac{1}{4}$ cup Parmesan cheese
1 cup half-and-half

- Scoop out tomatoes. Set upside down to drain for a few minutes. Put tomatoes in a baking dish and sprinkle with black pepper and basil. Slide into a 350° F oven for about five minutes. Watch them—don't let skins explode. Set aside.
- Melt butter in pan. Add garlic and zucchini and sauté quickly. Stir in half-and-half and cheese.
- Stuff mixture into tomato shells.

GREEN SALAD WITH MUSTARD VINAIGRETTE

Assorted salad greens

- Wash greens and set aside in a bowl.

Mustard Vinaigrette

3 tbsp. oil
1½ tbsp. tarragon vinegar

black pepper
2 tsp. Dijon-style mustard

- Whip ingredients together and toss with salad greens.

ASSORTED FRUITS

Not too many people in my family are dessert eaters, which is not to say we are saints, but we would just as soon go without. Since this is a picnic, an assortment of fruit would be fine and would satisfy anyone who simply had to eat more!

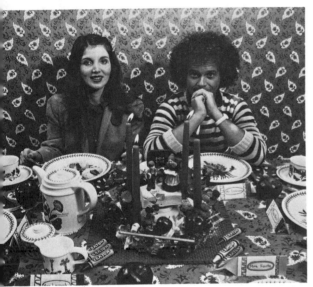

Mary Hoag

BACK-TO-SCHOOL TEA FOR TEACHERS

I held Teacher's Tea, and everyone had a great time.
Even though I have been teaching for thirteen years, I always get a special feeling when one of my kindergarteners hands me an apple!

⊷ MENU ⊷

Filled Apples
Apple Gelatin
"Easy As Pie" Apple Cake
Open-Face Sandwiches

Decorations

- centerpiece: straw wreath covered with artificial apples, bows, candles, pencils, and eucalyptus
- music box playing "School Days"
- pencil-shaped place cards
- crocheted apple pins.

FILLED APPLES

- For each apple, cut around the stem and save the top piece. Using a potato peeler, scrape most of the apple out from the middle. Discard seeds and leave enough apple near the skin so it has some body to it.
- Rinse the inside of the apple with lemon juice mixed with water to prevent browning. Keep the apple chunks in lemon water also while mixing ingredients.

Filling

apple chunks from one apple
¾ tbsp. mayonnaise
2 tbsp. plain yogurt

2 chopped dates
2 chopped walnuts

- Blend ingredients and fill apple.
- You can replace the top of the filled apple by pushing the top into a toothpick and sticking it back on the apple.

APPLE GELATIN

3 cups apple juice
2 packages unflavored gelatin

1 cup apple, shredded
1 banana, finely cut

- Heat the apple juice in a saucepan until it boils. Remove from heat.
- Dissolve gelatin into the apple juice. Chill until slightly thickened (about one hour).
- Add the shredded apple and the banana.
- Pour into a mold and chill until set.
- Yield: eight small servings.

"EASY AS PIE" APPLE CAKE

4 cups apple (4 apples, diced, unpeeled)
1 cup flour
1 cup whole wheat flour
½ cup wheat germ
2 eggs
½ cup sunflower seed oil
¾ cup honey

1 tsp. vanilla
1 tsp. cinnamon
½ tsp. allspice
1 tsp. salt substitute
3 tsp. baking powder
½ cup chopped walnuts

- Stir all ingredients until well blended. Pour into a 9" x 13" pan. Bake at 350° F for 45–55 minutes.

Frosting

1 8-oz. package imitation cream cheese, softened
1 cup confectioners' sugar

1 tsp. vanilla
1 tbsp. margarine, softened

- Mix frosting ingredients together and spread on cooled cake.

OPEN-FACE SANDWICHES

- Cut a plastic margarine lid into the shape of an apple. Then put this pattern on slices of thin-sliced whole wheat bread and cut around them with a knife.
- Top each apple-shaped piece of bread with a favorite filling—egg salad, tuna salad, or shrimp salad.

Fillings

- Egg Salad: Chop hard-boiled eggs and blend with plain yogurt. Top with paprika.
- Tuna Salad: Mix tuna with plain yogurt and pickle relish.
- Shrimp Salad: Mix cooked shrimp with mustard and yogurt.

To Decorate

- Stem: Slice bread crust thinly, put an inch on top of sandwich, and press to hold.
- Leaf: Cut a small slice of pickle and press on top next to stem.

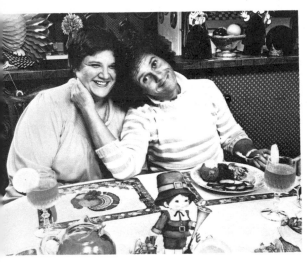

Lynn Thomas

HOLIDAY DINNER

My name is Lynn Thomas. I've lost over seventy-five pounds on the Richard Simmons Live-It.

I chose a Thanksgiving dinner as my contest entry. I love the warm, rich fall colors associated with the holiday. I also love the traditional foods served on that day, but I don't like the extra calories found in those foods. I have taken a traditional Thanksgiving meal and reduced the calorie count and fat content. At the same time I have tried to make the meal look festive and appetizing.

⊷ MENU* ⊷

HORS D'OEUVRES
Hot Mulled Cider
Stuffed Mushrooms
Garden Delight Relish Tray

APPETIZER
Fluted Fruit Cup

ENTREE
Turkey Italiano
Zesty Stuffed Baked Potatoes
Zucchini
Orange-Spiced Iced Tea

DESSERT
Pumpkin Custard

*These recipes serve eight.

HOT MULLED CIDER

4 cups apple cider (or apple juice)
8 whole allspice
5 whole cloves
1 tbsp. crushed cinnamon stick (see directions below)

1½ tsp. dried orange peel (see directions below)
1 small apple

For the crushed cinnamon: With a hammer, crush whole sticks of cinnamon until you have the desired amount.

For the dried orange peel: Using a zester, take several strips out of an orange peel. Set aside overnight. Break with fingers or chop with a knife until you have the desired amount.

- Make a bouquet garni of the allspice, cloves, cinnamon, and orange peel.
- Put cider into a covered saucepan. Bring to a boil. Lower heat, drop in bouquet garni, and let simmer twenty to thirty minutes.
- Cut small apple into crosswise slices. Remove any seeds. Garnish cider with one or two apple slices.

STUFFED MUSHROOMS

16 mushrooms
2 tbsp. bread crumbs
½ tsp. parsley flakes
1 tsp. onion, finely chopped

4 tsp. Parmesan cheese, grated
¼ tsp. garlic powder
1 tbsp. butter

- Remove stems from mushrooms. Chop stems and set aside. Place mushrooms, stem side down, under the broiler for three minutes.
- In a mixing bowl combine the chopped stems, bread crumbs, parsley, onion, two teaspoons Parmesan cheese, and garlic powder. Mix until blended.
- In a nonstick skillet melt butter. Add the bread crumb mixture to the butter in the skillet. Mix until butter is absorbed. Sauté mixture for three to five minutes.
- Stuff each mushroom cap with approximately half a teaspoon of the bread crumb mixture. Sprinkle the remaining Parmesan cheese over the top of the mushrooms. Place under the broiler for five minutes.

GARDEN DELIGHT RELISH TRAY

4 large stalks celery
2 carrots
1 cucumber
16 radishes
16 black olives

8 sweet midget pickles
endive
parsley
party toothpicks

Celery Curls

- Cut the celery stalks into three-inch pieces. Do not use the wide root ends. Using a paring knife, make one-inch deep cuts on both ends of celery piece until each end is shredded. Be careful not to cut through the middle. Chill in ice water until the ends curl.

Carrot Curls

- Peel, trim, and wash one carrot. Using a vegetable parer peel thin slices of carrot by starting at the top and running the parer the length of the carrot. Curl each thin strip around a finger. Slide off and secure with a toothpick. Chill in ice water until the toothpick is not needed to hold the curl.

Cucumber Rings

- Wash one cucumber but do not peel it. Using a corer remove seeds and pulp from the center of the cucumber. Using a zester remove a thin strip of cucumber peel, working lengthwise from one end to the other. Remove other strips in the same manner, spacing the strips evenly around the cucumber. Slice the cucumber crosswise into half-inch slices.

Radish Flowers

- Use eight radishes that are round in shape. Wash and trim. With a zester make a thin slice from the tops of the radishes almost to the bottoms. Be careful not to cut all the way through. Make five more slices that are evenly spaced around the radishes. Chill in ice water.

Radish Accordions

- Select eight radishes that are elongated. Wash and trim. Lay the radishes on their sides. Using a paring knife make eighth-inch wide slices, working from one end to the other. Do not make cuts all the way through the radishes. Chill in ice water.

Carrot Twist and Carrot Wheels

- Twist: Peel and wash one large carrot. With a fork score all sides of the carrot by drawing the tines of the fork down the length of the carrot. Using a spiral slicer slice half of the carrot. Bring both ends of the spiral together and secure with a toothpick. Chill in ice water.
- Wheels: Slice the rest of the carrot crosswise into eighth-inch slices.

The Tray

- On a serving tray make a bed of endive and parsley. In the center place the carrot twist. Place a radish flower on top of it. Place either a black or a green olive in each carrot curl. Secure with fancy toothpicks. Use fancy toothpicks for any remaining olives and for the pickles. Place all of the vegetables on the tray to make a pleasing arrangement.

FLUTED FRUIT CUP

4 small cantaloupes	1 cup purple grapes
1 small pineapple	2 kiwi fruit
1 cup white grapes	mint or parsley

- Using a food decorating tool, cut each cantaloupe in half so that it has a fluted edge. Scoop out seeds and discard. If the cantaloupe is not stable, cut a small slice from the bottom to make it flat.
- With a melon baller, make cantaloupe balls with as much of the cantaloupe as possible. Leave an eighth of an inch of melon around the edge and scoop out any extra pulp.
- Cut the pineapple into small chunks.
- In a large mixing bowl combine the cantaloupe balls, pineapple chunks, and grapes.
- Spoon the mixture into the cantaloupe shells.
- Peel the kiwi fruit and cut into sixteen slices. Use two slices for each fruit cup.
- Place the fruit cups on small plates. Garnish with a sprig of mint or parsley.
  NOTE: If the above fruits are not available, you can substitute any fruits that are in season for your area.

TURKEY ITALIANO

6 lbs. turkey breast, boned and skinned	8 tbsp. Parmesan cheese, grated
1½ cups tomato sauce (see Lynn's "That's Italian" tomato sauce recipe)	4 cloves garlic

- Cut garlic cloves in half. Rub garlic over turkey. Save garlic. Place turkey in a roasting pan that has a lid. Place garlic pieces on top of turkey. Cover and bake at 325° F. Allow twenty minutes per pound. (Weigh turkey after boning.)
- For the last fifteen minutes, uncover turkey and remove garlic. Continue baking until golden brown.
- When done, slice turkey, allowing three slices per person. Top each serving with three tablespoons tomato sauce and one tablespoon Parmesan cheese.

LYNN'S "THAT'S ITALIAN" TOMATO SAUCE

3–4 cloves garlic, chopped	2 8-oz. cans tomato puree
1–2 tbsp. onion, chopped	1 6-oz. can tomato paste
1 tbsp. olive oil	1 tbsp. oregano
water	

- In a large (six-quart) pot brown garlic and onion in olive oil. Add tomato puree, two cans full of water, and oregano. Bring to a slow boil and cook for twenty minutes. Add tomato paste. Stir until tomato paste dissolves. Add more water if sauce is too thick. Let sauce cool and simmer (uncovered) for four to five hours, stirring occasionally and adding water if needed.
  NOTE: Make the tomato sauce ahead of time. Reserve one and a half cups for the TURKEY ITALIANO and freeze the rest. Cooking the sauce for a long time is the secret to a good tomato sauce. It makes the sauce less acidic and easier to digest.

ZESTY STUFFED BAKED POTATOES

8 medium potatoes
1 8-oz. container plain nonfat yogurt
5 tbsp. nonfat dry milk solids
2½ tsp. lemon juice
1 tbsp. parsley flakes

1 tbsp. onion, minced
1 tsp. dill weed
½ cup low-fat milk
8 tbsp. Parmesan cheese, grated

- In a mixing bowl combine yogurt, dry milk solids, lemon juice, parsley flakes, minced onion, and dill weed. Blend well with a wire whisk.
- Refrigerate overnight.
- Bake potatoes for two hours at 325° F. Remove from oven.
- Cut an oblong hole in the top of each potato. Scoop out insides of potatoes and place in a large bowl.
- Combine potato pulp, yogurt mixture, milk, and seven tablespoons of Parmesan cheese. Mash.
- Spoon stuffing mixture into potato shells until they are almost full.
- Put remaining mixture in a pastry bag with a decorative shell tip on the end. Squeeze shells or stars to fill each potato.
- Sprinkle remaining Parmesan cheese over the top of the potatoes and return to the oven for ten to fifteen minutes.

ZUCCHINI

4 large zucchini

water

- Wash and trim zucchini. Slice into half-inch slices. Steam for ten minutes.

ORANGE-SPICED ICED TEA

3 Lipton Gentle Orange herbal tea bags
2 cups cold water

2 lemons

- In a small saucepan boil water. Add tea bags and steep for ten to fifteen minutes. Discard bags. Pour tea into a pitcher. Add enough cold water to make two quarts. Refrigerate several hours or overnight.
- Using a zester, remove a strip of lemon peel, working from top to bottom. Remove other strips in the same manner, spacing the strips evenly around the lemon. Slice crosswise into slices. Use slices to garnish each glass of tea.

PUMPKIN CUSTARD

2 cups canned pumpkin
2 cups low-fat milk
2 eggs, slightly beaten

4 tbsp. brown sugar
1 tsp. pumpkin pie spice
1 tsp. nutmeg

- Combine pumpkin, eggs, brown sugar, and pumpkin pie spice. Blend. Add milk and blend well.
- Pour into lightly greased custard cups. Sprinkle nutmeg on top. Place custard cups in a pan with one inch of water in it.
- Place this pan in the oven. Bake at 300° F for 1 hour.
- Refrigerate custard overnight.

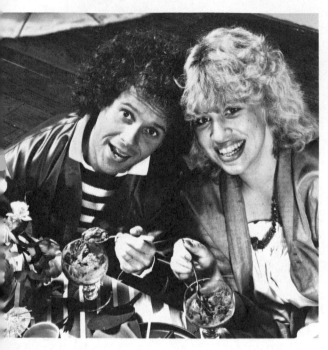

Troy Daigle

PARTICIPATORY PARTY

At my party we participated two ways. First, by exercising on a rebounder. Second, by helping our partners stir-fry the dinner.

⊰ MENU* ⊱

Almond Shrimp or Chicken Stir-Fry
Spinach Salad with Tomato Dill Dressing
Orange Pineapple Muffins
Fruit Porcupines
Rice
Raspberry Brandy Sherbet with Fortune Cookies

ALMOND SHRIMP OR CHICKEN STIR-FRY

3 lb. shrimp	1 green pepper
5 lb. chicken	3 cups bok choy
1 lb. mushrooms	1 pound snow peas
1 large head Chinese cabbage	1 pound bean sprouts
3 cups celery	4 oranges
4 small summer squash	1 cup almonds
2 large zucchini	rice
1 red pepper	

- Bone chicken and cut into small pieces (or clean shrimp).
- Slice squash, cabbage, and zucchini in long strips.
- Chop celery, mushrooms, peppers, and bok choy.
- Clean snow peas and bean sprouts.
- Peel oranges and divide into sections.

*These recipes serve twenty.

Each person picked a partner and together they cooked their dinner. They could pick any combination of vegetables and a choice of shrimp or chicken. Both partners had to agree on what went into the stir-fry. After the stir-fry was completed, we sprinkled a few almonds on top and served it with rice.

SPINACH SALAD WITH TOMATO DILL DRESSING

1 lb. spinach	1 cup radish sprouts
2 heads romaine lettuce	1 cup bamboo shoots
1 cup garden onions, chopped	1 cup water chestnuts
2 cups alfalfa sprouts	24 cherry tomatoes

- Combine all ingredients in a large bowl. Toss lightly.

Tomato Dill Dressing

1 cup wine vinegar	$\frac{1}{2}$ cup green onions, chopped
$\frac{1}{4}$ cup honey	$\frac{1}{2}$ cup freshly squeezed orange juice
$\frac{1}{2}$ cup safflower oil	1 tsp. dill weed
$\frac{3}{4}$ cup Italian tomatoes	

- Puree tomatoes and add honey. Mix well.
- Add remaining ingredients. Mix well.
- Refrigerate overnight in covered container.
- Shake well before serving.

ORANGE PINEAPPLE MUFFINS

5 tbsp. honey	2 cups whole wheat flour
2 eggs	1 cup unprocessed bran
$1\frac{1}{2}$ cups nonfat milk	$1\frac{1}{2}$ tsp. cinnamon
1 tsp. vanilla extract	1 tsp. nutmeg
$1\frac{1}{2}$ tsp. orange extract	$\frac{1}{2}$ tsp. allspice
1 cup crushed pineapple	$1\frac{1}{2}$ tsp. baking soda
$\frac{3}{4}$ cup freshly squeezed orange juice	

- Combine all wet ingredients EXCEPT orange juice.
- Combine all dry ingredients. Pour wet into dry ingredients slowly. Mix well by hand. Add orange juice. Mix well.
- Put mixture into muffin papers in a muffin pan. Bake at 375° F for 10–12 minutes or until they spring back when touched.
- Yield: fifty small muffins.

FRUIT PORCUPINES

watermelon	casaba melon
cantaloupe	pineapple
honeydew melon	kiwi fruit
cranshaw melon	strawberries

- Cube or slice fruit. Place into scooped pineapple shell.
- Decorate with Chinese umbrellas.

RASPBERRY BRANDY SHERBET WITH FORTUNE COOKIES

2 oz. crushed pineapple	1 cup pineapple juice
24 oz. frozen raspberries	6 cups nonfat milk
1 cup water	3 tsp. brandy extract
⅓ cup honey	2 tsp. vanilla extract

- Combine pineapple juice, honey, brandy extract, and vanilla extract. Set aside.
- Puree raspberries. Add to pineapple mixture. Mix well.
- Put milk and water into ice-cream freezer. Slowly add raspberry mixture. Mix well. Freeze until firm.
- Garnish with crushed pineapple and raspberries.
- Serve with fortune cookies.

Jan Ulrich

MOTHER-DAUGHTER BRUNCH

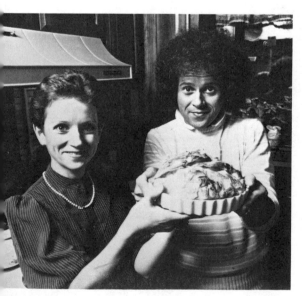

On the last day before my mother returned with my father to their home in Saudi Arabia, I gave a brunch to honor her and for all my friends' mothers.

My intention was to use all the seasonally fresh fruits and vegetables I could find. I used fresh zucchini, carrots, green onions, green beans, blueberries, strawberries, melons, peaches, cheeses, and shrimp.

I served this bounty of Northwest specialties buffet-style, with lovely summer flowers decorating the table and cool iced lemon tea for the beverage.

We had a lovely time, and the Moms were really delighted. In my recipes I used less salt, low-fat milk, and dairy products, and unflavored gelatin combined with natural fruit juices (instead of the commercial types). I made a serious attempt at using all fresh ingredients, and new recipes that can be completely or partially prepared ahead of time. This is especially useful for parents with active children who have little time for in-depth food preparation.

It was a wonderful excuse to have a party and to indirectly teach nutrition and good health. I loved it! Thank you for the experience.

—◂ **MENU** * ▸—

Zucchini-Carrot Garden Tart
Shrimp-Spinach "Caesar" Salad
Mixed Bean Vinaigrette
Jellied Layered Summer Fruit
"Seedy" Cracker Bread
Lemon Meringues
Iced Tea with Lemon
Coffee

ZUCCHINI-CARROT GARDEN TART

This recipe is a very handsome addition to a buffet table, and it is truly delicious. It is made with filo dough, which some people are scared to use, but with careful handling it is really easy.

4 small zucchini	2 tbsp. melted butter
4 medium carrots, shredded	$\frac{1}{2}$ tsp. salt
$\frac{1}{2}$ cup minced green onions	$\frac{1}{2}$ tsp. freshly ground pepper
2 cups low-fat (2%) cottage cheese	$\frac{1}{2}$ tsp. fresh dill
4 eggs (or equivalent in egg substitute)	8–10 sheets filo dough
$\frac{1}{4}$ cup milk	10-inch ceramic tart pan or heavy
$1\frac{1}{4}$ cup Parmesan or Romano cheese, freshly grated	heatproof pie plate

- Preheat oven to 375° F for ceramic pan or 350° F for a pie plate.
- Parboil quartered zucchini for five minutes, drain, and cool.
- Mix together zucchini, grated carrots, and green onions.
- Combine cottage cheese, eggs, milk, and seasonings.
- Blend cheese-egg mixture carefully into zucchini mixture and set aside. (It can be prepared up to six hours before and refrigerated.)
- Carefully unfold the filo, making certain the sheets are covered with a damp paper towel when they are not being used. Remove one sheet, leaving the remainder covered. Brush the sheet LIGHTLY with melted butter. Place the sheet in the bottom of the pie pan so that one short end reaches more than halfway across the pan and the other end overhangs the side. Repeat this procedure with five or six more sheets. Remember to LIGHTLY brush with butter as you overlap the sheets until the bottom is completely covered. Spoon cottage cheese–zucchini filling into the filo-lined pan. Smooth the top and sprinkle the grated cheese over the entire surface. Fold the overhanging dough over the filling, brush the remaining sheets of filo with melted butter (sparingly), and place on top to completely enclose the filling. Tuck the edges neatly in against the inside of the pan and brush the top with butter.
- Place the pie pan on a baking sheet and bake until the top of the tart is golden brown (forty to forty-five minutes). Cool on a wire rack about fifteen minutes before serving to allow the filling to set.
- Cut into wedges to serve.

*These recipes serve ten.

SHRIMP-SPINACH "CAESAR" SALAD

3 lemons
5 bunches of fresh spinach, rinsed and drained
½ cup celery, diced
2 large tomatoes
½ cup green onions, minced
1 clove garlic
½ tsp. salt
½ tsp. pepper, freshly ground

¼ tsp. mint
¼ tsp. oregano
½ cup raw sunflower seeds
½ pound fresh shrimp
¼ cup Parmesan or Romano cheese, freshly grated
1 tbsp. olive oil
4 oz. salad oil (preferably sunflower oil)
2 eggs, lightly beaten

- Oil the inside of your salad bowl with the olive oil, then rub the garlic into the oil. Set aside your seasoned salad bowl for thirty minutes to let the flavors mingle at room temperature.
- After you peel the tomatoes (by immersing in scalding water for thirty seconds), chop into large chunks and place with the diced celery. Then tear the spinach leaves and place lightly on top of the tomatoes and celery. At this point the salad can be refrigerated up to six hours ahead. Place a damp paper towel lightly over the spinach leaves and refrigerate.
- Prepare the following condiments for the salad: Mince the green onions and place in an airtight container. Grate the cheese and place in an airtight container. Rinse and drain the shrimp and place in an airtight container. Place all these condiments near the salad bowl in the refrigerator so you won't forget to add them when you're ready to serve.

Dressing

- In a glass jar squeeze the juice from the lemons, add the salad oil, eggs, freshly ground pepper, mint, oregano, and salt. Cover and shake again until well blended.
- Before serving toss the salad with all condiments and dressing. Sprinkle the top with sunflower seeds and serve.

MIXED BEAN VINAIGRETTE

1 16-oz. can of kidney beans, rinsed and drained
¾ cup celery, thinly sliced

1 small can garbanzo beans
1 cup fresh green beans, steamed

- Combine the beans and the celery in a large bowl and toss lightly.

Vinaigrette Dressing

¾ cup salad oil (sunflower)
¼ cup white vinegar
¼ tsp. paprika
¼ tsp. dry mustard
¼ tsp. cracked pepper

1 clove garlic, halved
¼ tsp. Worcestershire sauce
½ cup catsup
½ cup coconut, shredded

- Combine all the ingredients in a glass jar, cover tightly, and shake vigorously until well blended. NOTE: Keep garlic inside the bottle.
- Pour vinaigrette dressing over bean mixture and toss lightly until well blended.
- Chill in refrigerator at least twelve hours before serving.
- Sprinkle a garland of coconut over the salad before serving.

JELLIED LAYERED SUMMER FRUIT

4 envelopes unflavored gelatin	2 cups cantaloupe (or any melon)
3 cups lemonade	3 fresh peaches, sliced
2½ cups white wine	1 pt. blueberries
1 pt. fresh strawberries, hulled and washed	2 kiwi fruit
2 bananas	1 cup plain yogurt
1 cup seedless green grapes	12-cup glass salad bowl

- Sprinkle the gelatin over the lemonade in a saucepan. Let stand five minutes to soften. Place saucepan over low heat and stir constantly until the gelatin has dissolved (usually when the mixture has steam rising from it), then cool.
- Stir the wine into the gelatin mixture. Place in the refrigerator and allow the mixture to thicken to a jelly consistency.
- Place one cup of the lemon-wine jelly in the bottom of the glass bowl. Add a layer of jelly. Add layers of strawberries, grapes, blueberries, bananas, peaches, and melon, always alternating with the jelly.* Chill six hours or until set.
- Before serving, garnish with sliced kiwi and dollops of plain yogurt.

"SEEDY" CRACKER BREAD

This recipe calls for a food processor.

1 egg white, lightly beaten	½ tsp. salt
1¾ cups all-purpose flour	½ cup butter, cold
½ cup cornmeal	½ cup beer, flat
2 tbsp. sugar	2 tbsp. poppy seeds or sesame seeds
¼ tsp. baking soda	

- Place the flour, cornmeal, sugar, baking soda, and salt in the food processor. Cut the butter into six slices and add to the dry mixture. On PULSE speed, cut the butter into the flour mixture until it looks crumbly and stir in the beer. On PULSE speed again, mix until the dough forms a ball in the processor or until well blended.
- Preheat the oven to 375° F. Divide the dough into twenty-five small balls. On a lightly floured surface roll the balls into paper-thin circles (edges may be irregular) with a pancake turner. Place the circles one inch apart on an ungreased cookie sheet.
- Lightly brush the dough circles with egg white, then sprinkle with the seeds. With bottom of the pancake turner press the seeds firmly into the dough.
- Bake eight to ten minutes until lightly browned. With the turner remove the crackers to a wire rack to cool completely. Store in a tightly covered container.

*For the most aesthetic results, remember to layer with contrasting fruit colors.

LEMON MERINGUES

Meringue Shells

4   egg whites
1½ tsp. vanilla
½ tsp. lemon juice

1   cup sugar
½ cup graham cracker crumbs

- In a mixing bowl mix egg whites (preferably at room temperature), vanilla, and lemon juice. Beat into soft peaks. Slowly add the sugar, beating until very stiff peaks form and meringue is glossy. Fold in the graham cracker crumbs.
- Cover a baking sheet with heavy plain brown paper. Drop one-third cupfuls of meringue onto the paper, molding each into individual "bowls" with the back of a tablespoon. Bake at 275° F for one hour, then turn off the heat and leave the meringues in for one hour with the door closed. Let cool before filling.

Lemon Filling

2   cups pink lemonade
1   envelope unflavored gelatin

1   13-oz. can evaporated skim milk, chilled
1   lemon rind, grated

- Sprinkle the gelatin over the lemonade in a saucepan and let stand for five minutes to soften. Place over low heat and stir constantly until gelatin has dissolved and then cool. Whip the evaporated milk and add to the cooled gelatin mixture. Fold carefully and place in the refrigerator. Let stand for about one hour.
- When the filling is only partially set, fill individual shells, then lightly sprinkle with lemon rind. Before serving you may garnish with sliced strawberries, lemon twists, or blueberries for appeal.

Judy Jubb

DINNER PARTY

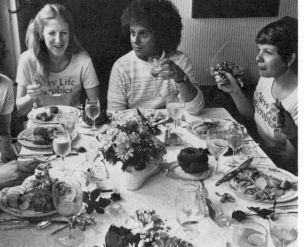

There was an 'de gang in a gym
That lifted and twisted to hymns
Then they all cooked a dinner
That was truly a winner
Now they're famous as well as slim trim.

The Rose-City Thighrockers is a group of eight women who fight rain, ice, and volcanic ash to exercise together three mornings a week. The music is loud, upbeat, and contemporary Christian. The exercise routines bring smiles to our faces and sweat to our bodies.

Following our "Oregon-ized Exercise" theme, our menu had predominantly Oregon specialties and we played a rousing round of musical chairs to determine the seating arrangement! Exercising together is a wonderful way to build relationships, and this contest has enhanced our time together.

Decorations

- spring flowers arranged on Nike aerobic dance shoes!
- name cards printed on a cutout of a Nike tennis shoe
- one long-stemmed red rose on each plate.

MENU*

APPETIZER
Skinny Artichokes

ENTREE
Crabby Sole
Twiggy Vegetables
Dilly Potatoes

DESSERT
Fresh Frozey Yogey

WINE
Tualitin Vineyards Chardonnay, 1979

SKINNY ARTICHOKES

4　artichokes	1　tbsp. Parmesan cheese
1　lb. cottage cheese	dash Worcestershire sauce
1　10-oz. package frozen spinach, thawed, with liquid squeezed out	

- Steam artichokes.
- Puree and heat four remaining ingredients in a saucepan over moderate heat.
- Remove center leaves and thistles from cooked artichokes. Spoon in pureed filling.

CRABBY SOLE

8　Petrale sole fillets	½　lb. crab meat
16　crab legs	

- Take fillets and add one tablespoon of crab meat to center. Place two crab legs extending out sides of sole and roll up. Place in 9″ x 12″ baking dish.

Sauce for Sole

3　8-oz. cans tomato sauce	2–3　cloves garlic, pressed
¼　cup white wine	½　cup Tillamook cheese, shredded

- Heat together all ingredients until warm.
- Pour over rolled sole and top with Tillamook cheese.
- Cook at 350° F for twenty-five to thirty minutes.

*These recipes serve eight.

TWIGGY VEGETABLES

2 medium-size zucchini	¼ cup vermouth
2 medium-size carrots	pinch of pepper, freshly ground
2 small onions	paprika
2 stalks celery	dill weed
1 tbsp. butter	garlic powder

- Julienne all vegetables.
- Sauté vegetables in electric frying pan with butter and vermouth.
- Sprinkle with a pinch of freshly ground pepper, then some paprika, dill weed, and garlic powder.
- Let vegetables soak for fifteen minutes without heat.
- Reheat to serve.

DILLY POTATOES

8 1½-inch diameter new potatoes	2 tsp. dill weed
1 tbsp. butter	

- Scrub potatoes and boil until tender.
- Heat butter with dill weed in frying pan, add potatoes, and roll them around until coated with butter and dill.

FRESH FROZEY YOGEY

4 plain Yoplait yogurt	8 tbsp. sliced almonds, toasted
2 pt. strawberries, fresh	6 oz. orange juice concentrate

- Marinate strawberries in orange juice concentrate for two to three hours.
- Drain and add to yogurt. Put in two tablespoons of reserved concentrate and blend in a blender.
- Place in freezer until slightly frozen.
- Whip and pour into eight parfait glasses.
- Top with one tablespoon of toasted almonds.